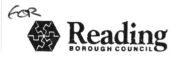

Post-Polio Syndrome

*A Guide for Polio Survivors
and Their Families*

JULIE K. SILVER, M.D.
FOREWORD BY LAURO S. HALSTEAD, M.D.

Yale University Press
New Haven & London

Set in Minion type by Keystone Typesetting, Inc.
Printed in the United States of America.

Library of Congress Cataloging-in-Publication Data
Silver, J. K. (Julie K.), 1965–
Post-polio syndrome : a guide for polio survivors and their families / Julie K. Silver ;
foreword by Lauro S. Halstead.
p.   cm.
Includes bibliographical references and index.
ISBN 0-300-08807-8 (cloth : alk. paper) — ISBN 0-300-08808-6 (pbk. : alk. paper)
1. Postpoliomyelitis syndrome.   I. Title.
RC180.1 .S56 2001
616.8'35—dc21   00-043801

A catalogue record for this book is available from the British Library.

The paper in this book meets the guidelines for permanence and durability of the
Committee on Production Guidelines for Book Longevity of the Council on Library
Resources.

10   9   8   7   6   5   4   3

To my beloved husband and children,
and to my favorite polio survivor—my mother

Contents

Foreword

Polio—like smallpox—is one of those ancient diseases that is destined to have a modern ending. According to the World Health Organization, acute paralytic poliomyelitis, after a run of many millennia, will be eliminated from the world not only in our lifetime but most likely in the next few years. In this country, the history of polio is much shorter. The main events were packed into a span of only thirty-nine years—barely two generations—beginning with the first major epidemic in 1916 (which was centered in New York City) and ending with the announcement on April 12, 1955, that the Salk vaccine was safe and effective. Since then, for most Americans, the epidemics have passed into oblivion, and polio no longer refers to a disease but to a vaccine. Yet for many thousands the legacy of our nation's brief rendezvous with polio is still very much a part of our personal histories and daily lives.

In the late 1970s, reports began to surface that people who had recovered from paralytic polio decades earlier were developing unexpected health problems such as excessive fatigue, pain in muscles and joints, and—most alarming of all—new muscle weakness. Because there was little in the modern medical literature about delayed neurological changes in polio survivors, the initial response of many physicians and other health-care workers was skepticism, if not outright ridicule. To complicate matters, this cluster of symptoms had no name. And without a name there was, in essence, no disease. Having a name—even if imprecise and misleading as to cause—helps establish an identity and an element of legitimacy. A name also makes it possible to begin the long journey from ignorance to understanding, and perhaps even to a cure. This journey finally began in the 1980s, when the many thousands of persons experiencing the late effects of polio started to attract the attention of the medical community. The term *Post-Polio Syndrome* (PPS) was coined.

Yet Post-Polio Syndrome was not a new disorder after all. Under a different name, the symptoms were first described in the French medical literature as far back as 1875; then, as often happens in medicine, they were forgotten. Over the next century, approximately thirty-five reports on post-polio weakness were published in the world's medical literature. Why these late effects of polio remained until recently an obscure and largely unexplored corner of medicine is unclear. Few diseases are as widely prevalent or have been as intensively investigated. Possibly because of the rapid and dramatic onset of symptoms, often followed by a near-miraculous recovery of function, polio was viewed primarily as a classic example of an acute viral illness. Most of the scientific energy and resources employed were directed at early management and prevention, with virtually no research into long-term sequelae or aftereffects. Medical textbooks classified paralytic polio as a *static* or *stable* neurological disease.

Fortunately, the early 1980s saw change. In May 1984 the first medical conference on PPS was held in Warm Springs, Georgia, to clarify causes and treatments and identify the major research questions. The subsequent years saw a marked increase in the attention focused on PPS by researchers and clinicians. The results were a more precise definition, a better understanding of possible causes, and more effective management. In 1994 the New York Academy of Sciences and the National Institutes of Health cosponsored another medical conference that culminated in the publication of a special issue of the *Annals of the New York Academy of Sciences* entitled "The Post-Polio Syndrome: Advances in the Pathogenesis and Treatment." Although much remains to be learned, that conference signaled acceptance of PPS by the medical establishment as a legitimate clinical entity. Polio survivors and their new problems had indeed come a long way.

However, for many of us the journey is far from over. Our polio disabilities, often compounded by aging and other health conditions, remain a daily struggle as our independence and quality of life continue to erode. On a broader level, we are like wounded veterans from some forgotten war whose presence has vanished from the national consciousness. Funding for desperately needed research is woefully inadequate, presenting a different kind of struggle with its own frustrations and disappointments, including the erosion of hope. There still is no diagnostic test for PPS, and the underlying causes remain ambiguous. While numerous treatments have been proposed, definitive therapies for most problems are unlikely for years to come.

In the meantime, our best recourse is improved management based on what we do know, which is exactly what Julie Silver prescribes in *Post-Polio Syndrome*. This book is much more than another skillful, comprehensive review of the literature dealing with the symptoms and treatment of the late effects of polio. It belongs to that small, select group of medical texts that is stylish, informative, and a pleasure to read. As Dr. Silver states in her preface, she wrote this book for a wide audience, including health-care professionals and friends and family members of persons who had polio years ago. While these groups will enjoy and profit from this volume, the greatest beneficiaries will be the polio survivors themselves. Another title for this volume could have been *Everything You Always Wanted to Know About Post-Polio, But Didn't Have an Expert to Ask*. Well, now you have one. You will meet her in these pages, which are crammed with up-to-date information and useful anecdotes designed to help prevent or minimize further disability and to improve the quality of your life.

I had the pleasure of working with Dr. Silver during her residency in Physical Medicine and Rehabilitation during the early 1990s, but her expertise with polio predated by many years our time in the Post-Polio Clinic in Washington, D.C. Although she never had the disease herself, she had the uncommon experience of growing up with polio; her mother, uncle, and grandfather all were polio survivors. I believe this background explains why she communicates a sense of comfort as well as competence. It is as though she has been diagnosing and treating polio problems all her life. But Dr. Silver is clearly more than a well-informed "polio doc." Her writing conveys a sense of commitment and affection for her patients, qualities to which I can attest from personal observation.

Finally, she writes about the importance of finding a physician who is both knowledgeable and sympathetic to the kinds of problems persons with polio are experiencing. Fortunately for her patients, she has both these qualities, a fact that helps to explain why she has such a busy practice and is so widely admired by patients and colleagues alike. Individuals who have Dr. Silver as their physician are truly fortunate. For those who cannot be treated by her personally, reading her book is the best alternative.

Lauro S. Halstead, M.D.

Preface

In the summer of 1946, my grandfather helped a neighbor build a patio. The next day he felt dreadful. In excruciating pain and unable to walk, he was hospitalized with paralytic polio. In addition to complete paralysis of his arms and legs, he had difficulty breathing and swallowing and used an iron lung for a brief period. Very shortly after my grandfather became ill, my mother and her younger brother also contracted polio. Fortunately, their cases were milder and they could be tended at home by my grandmother.

According to a family story, my grandfather was initially under the care of a compassionate young doctor, who unfortunately contracted polio himself—presumably from one of his patients. When I asked my grandfather shortly before his death in 1997 about this tale, he told me it was true. No one in my family is quite sure what happened to the young doctor, but apparently he died.

I am unable to pinpoint exactly when I became interested in polio. It seems to have always been a part of my life and my family history. When I was a child, my mother would tell me stories of what happened that summer of 1946. As in many polio families, there was little acknowledgment from my grandfather or grandmother of how dramatically polio altered their lives and the lives of their children. My grandfather eventually learned to walk with a long leg brace and crutches, but he was out of work for more than a year. He was thankful that his company had held his job as a chemical engineer, but he had to move to an office in a separate building (away from his peers) because of problems with accessibility. Whether because of the physical distance between my grandfather and his coworkers, his disability, or some other reason, he never advanced in his profession at the rate he had prior to becoming ill. As for my mother and her brother, within weeks to months of contracting polio they recovered with few residual effects. They went on with their lives as though nothing unusual had happened. But of course it had.

I suppose I always knew that there was more to this story. Surely a disease such as polio could not have swept through my family leaving my grandfather permanently disabled without having profound lasting effects. So my first interest in polio was really in what happened to the people who were affected and their loved ones (in my family and in other families). How did they overcome this dread disease, or did they? As I got older and began to study medicine, my interest in these people and their lives expanded to include the practical aspects of treating medical problems that arose in polio survivors as they aged. I gained invaluable experience and insight when I had the opportunity to work with Dr. Lauro Halstead at the Post-Polio Clinic (National Rehabilitation Hospital) in Washington, D.C.

When I started my own practice, I was discouraged by the general lack of support of the medical community for polio survivors. I have found polio survivors themselves to be hungry for information that will help them live their lives to the fullest. In fact, my very first talk on polio was given to a standing-room-only crowd. Since then I have traveled quite extensively, speaking to polio survivors and their loved ones as well as to health-care professionals. People often ask me for more information and for resources on aging with polio, and that is the origin of this book. I wanted to write a comprehensive volume that would help prevent further disability in polio survivors as they age. Consequently, this book was written to benefit polio survivors and their loved ones. It was also written for health-care providers who are interested in medical issues germane to aging with polio. Many of the examples I use derive from my own experiences in treating polio survivors. Although the names and identifying characteristics of the people involved have been changed in order to protect their privacy, their stories are factual and invaluable.

If I have done my job well, by the time you finish reading this book, you too will be better able to prevent further disability in your own life or in the lives of polio survivors whose paths cross yours.

* * *

There are many people to whom I am grateful for their help in putting this book together. First and foremost is my husband, Jim, who is a constant source of encouragement and advice. Next is the chairman of my department (Physical Medicine and Rehabilitation) at Harvard Medical School, Walter Frontera, who has unfailingly supported me in all of my academic endeavors and who was instrumental in helping me obtain a grant in order to complete this book. Lauro Halstead—physician, polio survivor, and leading expert on Post-Polio Syndrome—has been my teacher, mentor, and colleague for many years. I am profoundly grateful for his role in my professional life. Kristin Wainwright, my literary agent, and Jean Thomson Black, my editor at Yale University Press, worked both with me and with each other to bring this book from conception to completion. Nancy Tanner and Kari Hastings, of the research and development office at Spaulding Rehabilitation Hospital in Boston, helped tremendously with manuscript preparation and research, respectively. Terry O'Brien and Terry Cucuzza, librarians at that hospital, were instrumental in locating books and articles for me. Carol Foxman, a research librarian at the Massachusetts General Hospital, did most of the literature searches for this book.

In order to represent the views of medical experts who are

knowledgeable about polio and Post-Polio Syndrome, I asked a number of health-care providers to review the chapters.

• The following people were extraordinarily generous with their time, and their comments have made this a far better book: Dorothy Aiello, Ali Buckley, Jane Clark, Maria Cole, Suzanne Dagesse, Robert Drillio, Walter Frontera, Lauro Halstead, Charlie Henry, Sally Johnson, Lisa Krivickas, Raul Laguarda, Ellen Marcus, Eddie Phillips, and Eileen Winston.

• Hugh Gallagher, an award-winning writer and a polio survivor, was kind enough to review several chapters, as was Elaine Burns, who is president of the Greater Boston Post-Polio Society. Heidi Raine, my friend and fellow writer, was not intimately familiar with polio and thus gave me a fresh perspective.

• The members of the Assistive Technology Department at Spaulding Rehabilitation Hospital were enormously helpful to me on several occasions.

• A number of other people helped in various ways as I was researching, writing, and preparing the manuscript for this book. My heartfelt thanks go out to all of these people for their time, expertise, and encouragement. This book would not have been possible without them.

Post-Polio

Syndrome

CHAPTER 1

Polio—A Look Back

Polio is spectacular, the way it strikes, the way it kills, the way it leaves its
trademark.
—ROBERT F. HALL, *Through the Storm*

There has never been a disease quite like polio. Unique in ways that
defy explanation, it has created a legacy of shattered lives that continues to this day.

Poliomyelitis is an ancient disease, with references dating back to
the Old Testament. In 1500 B.C., an Egyptian stone carving showed a
priest leaning on a staff—one leg smaller and shorter than the other,
his foot pointed in the manner characteristic of polio. In the 1700s, a
British physician named Michael Underwood formally described
polio after numerous outbreaks. Although Dr. Underwood did not
officially name the disease, he described it as a "debility" of the lower
extremities.[1] Prior to the twentieth century, polio occurred spo-
radically and affected relatively few people. Thus, descriptions and
understanding of the disease were quite limited.

The situation changed dramatically when epidemics swept across
the United States and many other parts of the world in the late 1800s.
The first were described in Scandinavian towns in the 1880s and
1890s. Then, in 1894, a small town in Vermont reported forty-four
cases of paralytic polio. The dreadful shift from an endemic disease,
which occurred infrequently and was overshadowed by many other
contagious diseases such as smallpox and diphtheria, to a disease of

epidemic proportions, which eventually killed and maimed millions of people, is remarkable. In less than a decade, polio would become a menacing disease that attacked hordes of children and adults with a vengeance unlike that of any other illness. In her eloquent memoir entitled *In the Shadow of Polio*, Kathryn Black describes the alarming way in which polio could infect an individual and be almost unnoticed, and in another person seriously maim or even kill. Black writes: "Polio varies widely not only in its intensity but in its lasting effects. Children can hover near death fully paralyzed and recover completely, or they can be left with paralysis ranging from the inconvenient to the tragic."[2]

Polio's transformation to an epidemic that topped the country's social and political agendas in the first half of the twentieth century was paradoxically due in large part to technological advances. Naomi Rogers, in *Dirt and Disease*, describes how the period from 1890 to 1920 (the Progressive Era) brought about the relatively new concept that germs are transmitted in unsanitary conditions. This germ theory prompted authorities at all levels to encourage greater cleanliness, which was to be manifested in a variety of ways from improved personal hygiene to more sanitary water sources. Rogers notes that this effort had social and political implications as well: "As health officials guarded the community's health by keeping food, water, and streets clean, disease became a sign of individual irresponsibility, a failure to carry out the well understood rules of modern hygiene."[3] Sadly, while the improvements in sanitation markedly reduced many of society's former ills, it unpredictably allowed polio to flourish. The notion was well ingrained that if people bathed regularly, washed their hands, kept their homes clean, and treated their sewage, they would be safe from germs and disease. How could it be that polio did not play by the rules? Edward Tenner summarizes the counterintuitive way in which the polio epidemics are thought to have evolved: "As early as the 1920s and 1930s, epidemiologists were finding that the crusade for cleanliness at the beginning of the century, far from combating polio, was promoting it. When all infants acquired the virus in the first days of their lives, while still protected by antibodies from their mothers' blood, paralysis was almost unknown. Epidemics became most severe where standards of plumbing and cleanliness were highest. There, young people were first exposed to the virus long after the end of maternal immunity."[4]

This theory is now widely accepted. If a child is exposed to the polio virus in infancy while the mother's antibodies are still present, the child is able to produce his or her own antibodies without ever contracting the disease. It is known that, years ago, individuals infected with the polio virus would shed the virus in their stools. Water supplies contaminated with that fecal material would provide the early exposure babies needed in order to develop a natural immunity to polio. When sewage treatment plants became widely available, the polio virus was largely eradicated from the usual sources that provided infants with this exposure. Thus, the polio epidemics followed a pattern of primarily occurring in areas of socioeconomic privilege, where sanitation was widely available.

During the epidemic years, when little was initially known about the transmission of polio, theories abounded. Moreover, as with any serious illness in which a cure or vaccine seems unlikely in the near future, prevention became the focus. From all avenues came theories of how to prevent polio; they ranged from the outrageous to the implausible to the possible. Fear of the unknown fueled a near-panic state. Many parents guarded their children during the spring and summer months, when polio was most likely to occur. There are many tales of mothers allowing their children out only after dark, or only with gloves on their hands. Sometimes children were sent away to summer camps in the hope that a remote region would be safer. Others were kept home, with vacations canceled for fear that traveling would expose children to the illness. They were cautioned not to drink from fountains. Swimming, then the only way to cool off during the hot summer months, was frequently forbidden. One mother told me she kept her three young sons in the house the entire summer and never once let them go outdoors during a polio epidemic in her Massachusetts town. Here is what it was like during the early epidemic years.

> The mothers are so afraid that most of them will not even let the children enter the streets, and some will not even have a window open. In one house the only window was not only shut, but the cracks were stuffed with rags so that "the disease" could not come in. The babies had no clothes on, and were so wet and hot they looked as though they had been dipped in oil, and the flies were sticking all over them. I had to tell the mother I would get the Board of Health after her to make her open the window, and now if any of the children do get infantile paralysis, she will feel that I killed them. I do not wonder they are afraid. I went to see one family about four p.m. Friday. The baby was not well and the doctor was coming. When I returned Monday morning there were three little hearses before the door; all her children had been swept away in that short time. The mothers are hiding their children rather than give them up.[5]

Because no one knew how polio was transmitted, people legitimately were afraid to be around anyone who had recently contracted the disease. I have thought a lot about the young doctor mentioned earlier who cared for my grandfather when he had polio. In the middle of my grandfather's hospital stay, this doctor reportedly contracted polio himself and died. Polio survivors have told of being placed in isolation for fear they would spread the disease. Children were frequently taken from their homes and forced to fend for themselves in hospital rooms with only the most perfunctory nursing care. Many polio survivors have haunting memories of feeling abandoned by their parents, who either were not allowed to visit their children at all or were permitted only brief visits, sometimes from behind a curtain or glass window. Further devastating to these children was the fact that often all of their possessions were burned or discarded, for fear that those might somehow spread the disease. Unfortunately, many polio survivors continue to live with the psychological wounds that were inflicted when they were sick and in pain, and their familiar world instantaneously disappeared as they were literally whisked out of their parents' arms and placed in a sterile hospital bed.

For many polio survivors, looking back is a painful process. Perhaps because the psychological wounds never healed as fully as the physical ones. The ignorance and fear that ran rampant were powerful forces in determining how individuals infected with the polio virus would be medically treated. Admittedly, it is easy to look back and criticize the manner in which many polio survivors were treated; yet the fact remains that their medical care was crude, based on ignorance, and in some instances downright harmful. It is only retrospectively that we know how traumatized polio survivors were, not from the disease itself or from the resulting disability, but from the way they were treated in a "safe" hospital environment. We now know that although many survivors were cared for at home by loving parents, or in hospitals by compassionate doctors and nurses, others were not so fortunate. Some were abused, and those who were children at the time of their illness were the most vulnerable. Frank accounts of sexual and physical abuse have been reported by polio survivors who have found the courage to confront these painful issues. The following excerpt is from *A Summer Plague:*

> The nursing care was just appalling. I was largely incontinent unless I had someone there to give me a bedpan or a bottle the moment I needed it, because I couldn't move at all. However I was strapped in the bed, and strapping in the bed was used as a punishment if you wet the bed or shit yourself or whatever. Looking back now, I can hardly believe that young kids, some of whom couldn't have been more than a year old, were smacked for wetting themselves.

I had difficulty swallowing and breathing because I'd had bulbar polio, but when I didn't want my food they used to hold my nose and stuff greens down my throat—greens not being my favourite thing. . . . I was put out in the sun at one stage and just left there, and I ended up with a sunburned face, quite severe sunburn. That was another way of punishing you—roll out on the bed and leave you there in the sun. These are things that are difficult to pin down if you're trying to accuse somebody, but when you're experiencing them you know. Also things like leaving me unattended in the bath—I mean, I could've drowned because I couldn't hold myself up; I was still virtually paralyzed.[6]

Regardless of whether an individual had a nurturing experience or was severely abused during the acute illness, polio survivors en masse were encouraged to get on with their lives and get back to "normal." Marc Shell, a polio survivor and professor of comparative literature at Harvard University, teaches a course on the history of paralysis. He mentioned to me that as he read the essays of polio survivors he detected strong feelings of denial (which come across as a rather peculiar optimism) permeating the memoirs. In part, these feelings may reflect societal expectations that the survivors adopted and incorporated into their own psychological belief systems.

One recurrent theme is that polio was actually a blessing in disguise and helped change the life course of the individual in a positive manner. Dr. Richard Owen, who has done substantial research on the topic of Post-Polio Syndrome, describes how polio changed his life: "Instead of sports and fighting, I started to put my energies into my studies. I could no longer compete on the athletic field, but I could compete in the classroom. Therefore, I think polio made me into more of a scholar after my first twelve years of being very unscholarly. It made me want to do better than other people in school because I wanted to prove myself. If I hadn't had polio, I probably wouldn't have gone to medical school, and I have no idea what else I might have done for a career."[7]

Dr. Lauro Halstead, a polio survivor and a world-renowned expert on PPS, explains how denial and the ability to persevere both helped and hindered him:

> My own experience taught me the mixed blessings of denial. I had recovered and yet did not feel disabled; nor did I grieve. Even though my right arm remained largely paralyzed, I did not think of myself as handicapped. That kind of magical thinking was apparently not unusual among polio patients. Our desperate struggle to survive, work hard, and excel led to a series of negative lessons that I believe many of us polios learned, whether we realized it or not. We developed strong denial systems that have kept many of us distanced from the voices of our bodies. We are horrified and outraged at the possibility of being sick again, and we don't want to know that what we worked so hard to achieve might be lost. I believe this helps explain why so many polios are reluctant to seek help when they develop weakness in both themselves and others. By walling themselves up, they thus isolate from new disasters and become detached from their own feelings.[8]

Dr. Halstead's words are quoted from a chapter he wrote, titled "The Lessons and Legacies of Polio." I routinely distribute this chapter with other polio materials to patients and to polio survivors who attend my lectures. Time and time again, people have come back to me and said that Halstead's words resonate with their own unresolved feelings of denial. Interestingly, polio survivors as a group tend to be very intelligent, hardworking, and successful. The denial mechanisms that are so deeply rooted in their past have served them well in terms of their accomplishments. However, these same denial mechanisms may deter some of them from seeking help when physical or psychological healing is a necessity.

Perhaps the most magnificent lessons in the art of denial came from Franklin Delano Roosevelt. Wildly successful in his professional life, FDR was unable to walk even a step without the assistance of bodyguards who would literally carry him. In a moving portrait of the former president, entitled *FDR's Splendid Deception,* award-winning author Hugh Gallagher describes the fantastic illusion Roosevelt maintained in order to deny his disability: "Although there are over thirty-five thousand still photographs of FDR at the Presidential Library, there are only two of the man seated in his wheelchair. No newsreels show him being lifted, carried, or pushed in his chair . . . This was not by accident. It was the result of a careful strategy of the President. The strategy served to minimize the extent of his handicap, to make it unnoticed when possible and palatable when it was noticed. The strategy was eminently successful, but it required substantial physical effort, ingenuity, and bravado. This was FDR's splendid deception."[9]

In order to truly appreciate the President's disguise of his disability, consider the fact that he "was the only person in the recorded history of mankind who was chosen as a leader by his people even though he could not walk or stand without help."[10] During FDR's incumbency, the media did not scrutinize politicians in the same manner as today. Roosevelt carefully honed his image, and the media went along with it. Known for founding Warm Springs in Georgia, a legendary retreat with healing thermal springs and mud baths where polio survivors could convalesce, and for helping to organize the National Foundation for Infantile Paralysis (NFIP), which would later be known as the March of Dimes, FDR was revered by polio survivors and by society in general. But his eldest son, James, remembers a different man from the one the public knew:

> It's easy to look back now and say that he contracted polio and learned to live with it; that with the encouragement of Louis Howe, Eleanor Roosevelt paved the path for Franklin Roosevelt's return to politics over the opposition of [his mother] Sara Roosevelt; that he swiftly ascended to the governor's chair and finally to the presidency. But that isn't fair to father. It was more than three years before he hobbled briefly back into the spotlight, eight years before he became governor and twelve years

before he became president. The suffering and struggling of all those days, weeks, months and years are not to be taken lightly. I was thirteen when he was stricken and twenty-five when he became president. I grew up with his suffering and struggling.[11]

Almost certainly FDR's splendid deception and denial of his limitations allowed him to accomplish what few men, disabled *or* able-bodied, have ever been able to do. Warm Springs became a haven for polio survivors that to this day functions as a rehabilitation facility for people with many kinds of illnesses and injuries. The March of Dimes, the most popular charity of its time, raised money to essentially pay for the medical care of anyone who became infected with polio. A national call went out to leave one's porch lights on if the homeowners were willing to donate dimes to the mothers who went from door to door collecting for the cause. This practice became so lucrative that, at a time when medical insurance was relatively unknown, people who did not have polio but had some of the same symptoms (fever, muscle pain, and the like) occasionally were given the diagnosis of polio simply to ensure that their medical bills would be paid. There are individuals who have believed their entire lives that they were afflicted with polio, when in fact they never had the disease at all. Although these cases are uncommon, they do exist because of the sheer power and financial support that the March of Dimes was able to generate.

The March of Dimes was also instrumental in funding scientific research, particularly that directed at finding a vaccine to prevent polio. In 1908 Karl Landsteiner and his assistant, Erwin Popper, identified the causative agent in polio as a virus. Despite this monumental step, it would be nearly half a century before a vaccine was developed. During this time many scientists all over the world participated in the development of both treatment of those who were afflicted with polio and prevention for those who were not.[12]

The best-known researchers in the polio vaccine effort are two men who were successful in producing different vaccines—Jonas Salk and Arthur Sabin. Salk developed the first polio vaccine in the early 1950s, and it was licensed for general use in 1955. It was a killed vaccine (also known as an inactivated polio vaccine) and was considered quite safe because it could not cause new cases of polio. Sabin's vaccine, on the other hand, was a live (attenuated) vaccine that came into general use in 1962. Although both vaccines had advantages and disadvantages, Sabin's was ultimately considered superior. There are still many advocates of the Salk vaccine, because of the rare instances in which an individual who is given the Sabin vaccine actually develops polio from the vaccine itself. Undeniably, both men made enormous contributions to the prevention of polio; however, they were known to have disliked each other intensely. Part of polio's legacy is the bitter rivalry between Salk and Sabin.

Polio was the preeminent social, political, and health issue of the first half of the twentieth century. Although there was terrific rejoicing when the Salk vaccine was first introduced, it appeared against a backdrop of families grieving for loved ones who had been too late to receive the vaccine and had succumbed to polio. Further, scientists were engaged in acrimonious political struggles that would forever mar the two men's scientific contributions. The vaccines were introduced after other vaccines had been tried and had failed either because they were unable to prevent polio infection when someone was exposed, or in some tragic cases infected the person with the disease at the time of vaccination.

Henry Hampton, the documentarian whose film *Eyes on the Prize* became the nonfiction standard for chronicling the civil rights movement, told me that when he was fifteen years old his father, who was a physician, withheld the polio vaccine from his own children in an attempt to be certain it was safe. It was a decision he would later regret. Hampton recalled, "My father had the vaccine sitting in his office when I contracted polio." Desperately ill for weeks, Henry eventually survived the acute illness but never walked again unaided.

Just prior to the introduction of the Salk vaccine, the polio epidemic was at its peak, with nearly sixty thousand cases reported in 1952. In 1957, the first year in which ample supplies of the vaccine were available, the number of reported cases dropped to less than six thousand. The last reported case of the wild polio virus in the United States was in 1979, and the World Health Organization (WHO) is close to making polio extinct worldwide. After the initial vaccinations were carried out, polio declined so rapidly that the organizations that had supported its research, treatment, and ultimately prevention, needed to either disband or find another focus. Polio survivors had moved on with their lives, and the March of Dimes too moved on to other charitable work, including funding research to fight birth defects in children.

Although no one disputes that the current work of the March of Dimes is worthwhile, many polio survivors and their families feel abandoned by an organization that was once their lifeline. Now that the majority of polio survivors are experiencing new health problems many years after their initial infection, few resources are available to fund research and treatment for what is commonly known as Post-Polio Syndrome (PPS). Consequently, when the early reports of PPS surfaced in the late 1970s and early 1980s, polio survivors banded together and formed a large network of support groups in order to disseminate information about PPS, offer support to survivors, and sometimes lobby for research and treatment funding.

There are also a number of dedicated doctors, scientists, and other health-care providers who are working on research and treatment options that will help polio survivors as they age—regardless of whether they have PPS. Their work is the subject of this book.

CHAPTER 2

Post-Polio Syndrome

With the advent of the polio vaccines, the country's obsession with the disease ended. The vaccines were effective not only in eliminating polio but also in erasing its prominence on political and health-care agendas. In an amazingly short time, polio was obliterated as completely as if it had never existed. Polio survivors moved on with their lives, the March of Dimes went on to fight birth defects, and politicians promoted other causes. Even medical doctors, if they studied it at all, learned about polio as a historical footnote. Polio was so thoroughly expunged from our national consciousness that it did not seem possible that the nightmares of years gone by could be resurrected.

But in fact, the unimaginable happened. After a long dormant period, during which the vaccines prevented new cases of acute polio, in the late 1970s and early 1980s it became clear that vestiges of the virus had returned to haunt the very people who had survived its initial onslaught. This did not happen in the dramatic, catastrophic way in which polio had appeared in the past, but in a more insidious and persistent fashion. With increasing frequency, polio survivors began reporting new problems that bore a remarkable resemblance to symptoms they had experienced at the onset of the disease decades ago. At first these odd complaints were attributed to a variety of other maladies, including benevolent malingering. As time went on, and more and more polio survivors described a nearly identical set of symptoms, the realization took hold that perhaps these new manifestations were somehow related to the original polio infection. The characteristic symptoms were described in various ways as post-polio sequelae, the late effects of polio, and post-polio muscular atrophy. The term used throughout this book, Post-Polio Syndrome (PPS), is today the common name used to describe these symptoms.

Acute Poliomyelitis and Its Relation to Post-Polio Syndrome

Polio is caused by a virus and generally presents with fever, sore throat, diarrhea, and vomiting caused by the virus's invasion of the gastrointestinal tract. In fewer than 5 percent of polio cases, the virus actually invades the spinal cord and brain, which may result in paralysis and breathing and swallowing problems. The most severely affected individuals died—generally from bulbar polio, which paralyzes the muscles that control breathing and swallowing. Fortunately, the majority of people who had paralytic polio survived the disease and recovered at least partially from the point at which they were sickest.

The initial polio was highly unpredictable in that some who were severely paralyzed appeared to recover almost completely, while others who had less paralysis during the acute phase also experienced less recovery, which resulted in a more significant disability. Lauro Halstead's book *Managing Post-Polio* describes four stages of polio.[1] The first is the acute febrile illness in which the paralysis is most prominent. Generally in a matter of days, the individual's temperature returns to normal and the second stage begins. This period of convalescence or recovery may last from weeks to years, depending on the individual's age and the extent of the initial paralysis. Children who had extensive paralysis seem to take the longest to recover. Stated another way, children with extensive paralysis have the opportunity to improve for a much longer period than their adult counterparts, who enter the third stage more quickly. Stage three begins rather indeterminately when the individual reaches a level of maximal recovery. It is described as the stage of stable disability or chronicity, in which polio survivors spend most of their lives. Stage four, Post-Polio Syndrome, is experienced by a large number of polio survivors, but not all. It involves new medical problems that are related to having had polio in the past.

Post-Polio Syndrome is characterized by new symptoms that occur in people with a history of polio after a long period of stability (generally at least fifteen to twenty years) in which whatever strength they had remained unchanged. Frequently, the most prominent and alarming symptom of PPS is new weakness, either in a limb that was known to be involved in the acute illness or in a limb that was not thought to have been affected. This new weakness often heralds a more pronounced level of disability in polio survivors who believed that the worst was over. Some polio survivors are so taken aback by these symptoms that they do not seek treatment until years after the initial manifestations of PPS. In some instances, individuals simply deny that they are having new problems until their condition becomes so pronounced that denial is no longer possible. For other persons, a lack of understanding keeps them from seeking the medical care they need. Still other polio survivors, expert at managing adversity, may genuinely be unaware that anything out of the ordinary is occurring.

Sometimes the symptoms are so subtle that the only way to measure them is by taking a careful history that spans many years. A typical scenario is that of John Young.

As a young man, John was able to climb stairs uneventfully as long as there was a single railing. Thinking back, he recalls that ten years ago he began to avoid stairs unless they had a double railing. Five years ago, he began to avoid stairs altogether, and at this point he cannot go up stairs at all—even in an emergency situation. John may not have noticed any changes in strength from week to week; yet clearly there has been a dramatic decrease in his strength, which has led to an increased level of disability over the past decade.

The polio survivors who are used to being self-reliant may take new symptoms (such as weakness) for granted and simply adjust to a greater level of disability. Unfortunately, even the most motivated polio survivors can become discouraged when they finally do seek out medical treatment. They lament, rightfully, that they often know more than their doctors about PPS. Those who are discouraged may not persevere long enough to find polio experts who can intervene and provide help. Others are mistakenly convinced that if they give their doctors enough literature on PPS, these physicians will suddenly become experts and will be able to heal them.

Understanding Post-Polio Syndrome

Post-Polio Syndrome experiences the general lack of understanding that is characteristic of many syndromes. Its precise cause is poorly understood; probably it is several simultaneous elements. This is termed *multifactorial,* in that many factors are influencing the disease process. In PPS these elements include normal aging, in combination with accelerated aging of nerves that were injured by the initial polio. Another major factor is likely the overuse of nerves and muscles that are trying to do the same amount of work with fewer resources. I sometimes use the example of a construction crew that has lost several of its workers. This crew, which now consists of fewer workers but still has the same house to build by the same deadline, must work harder in order to accomplish the task. As the house progresses, more workers drop out because of fatigue and injury. Now the remaining crew is really at a disadvantage and simply cannot complete the task at the same rate or with the same level of skill. The nerves of polio survivors are the construction crew. In most cases, more than 95 percent were injured during the initial polio.[2] Many nerves died, and the remaining ones had to do their own work plus the work of those that died, in order to power the muscles of the body. Over the years, some of the surviving nerve cells just were not up to the task; when they dropped out, the remaining nerve cells did the best they could to compensate.

A syndrome is a collection of symptoms that characteristically occur together. By definition, a syndrome has no single test to identify it. Thus, it is attributed to someone only if they meet specific criteria established by the medical community, and only after all other reasonable (and testable) conditions have been eliminated as possibilities. For diagnosis of any syndrome, the following must occur: (1) an individual must present with specific symptoms, (2) all other possible causes for these symptoms must have been ruled out, and (3) the individual must meet the criteria established for diagnosis of the syndrome.

Because syndromes do not have specific tests that can unquestionably identify them, they are subject to interpretation. Often their validity is challenged within the medical community. PPS is no exception. Although most doctors believe that PPS exists, a few do not. Generally it is inexperienced health-care providers, unfamiliar with treating polio survivors, who dismiss the syndrome. Those of us who routinely participate in the care of polio survivors have no doubt that PPS is real.

Not surprisingly, the ability to diagnose PPS requires a physician to have extensive experience in treating polio survivors in order to know which symptoms may potentially be attributed to PPS rather than some other illness. The diagnosing physician must adhere strictly to the rules stated above for diagnosing any syndrome and must also be familiar with the criteria used to diagnose PPS.

Diagnosing Post-Polio Syndrome

STEP 1. EVALUATING THE SYMPTOMS

Post-Polio Syndrome is a neurological illness. For it to be named as the diagnosis, the symptoms an individual presents with must be consistent with those that are described as the syndrome. One does not need to have all of the manifestations listed below; however, if a patient complains of symptoms that are *not* listed, other diagnoses should be considered. Some of the symptoms are weighted more heavily than others, and new weakness—the sine qua non—is the most important criterion. The symptoms consistent with the diagnosis of PPS include the following:

- New weakness
- Unaccustomed fatigue
- Muscular pain
- New swallowing problems
- New respiratory problems
- Cold intolerance
- New muscle atrophy

STEP 2. ELIMINATION OF ALL OTHER POSSIBLE ILLNESSES

It is imperative to understand that PPS is a *diagnosis of exclusion*. In other words, the diagnosis of PPS is assigned only after other diagnoses have been excluded. In reality, it is impractical to test for all illnesses that may cause the symptoms described above. However, a responsible doctor will consider alternative diagnoses that may produce the same manifestations as PPS. The treating physician should perform an appropriate level of investigation for an alternative diagnosis by taking a careful history and conducting a thorough physical examination. Subsequent tests should be done with the intention of ruling out any disease that may be positively identified by a particular test and any disease in which treatment would differ from that of PPS.

STEP 3. MEETING THE CRITERIA FOR THE DIAGNOSIS
OF POST-POLIO SYNDROME

If Steps 1 and 2 have been completed and an individual has symptoms consistent with those described in PPS (and no other cause for the symptoms is determined), then the final step is to make certain the individual meets the criteria (as determined by the medical community) for PPS. Those criteria are as follows:

1. An individual must have a known history of polio. Documentation by electromyographic study (EMG) is generally recommended.
2. The individual must have had some improvement in strength following the initial paralysis.
3. There must have been a period of stability (at least one or two decades) in which the individual had no new symptoms.
4. The individual must present with new symptoms that are consistent with PPS and not attributable to some other disease.

Although these criteria are the accepted medical standard, recently individuals with a history of what was thought to be nonparalytic polio have been diagnosed with PPS.[3] Additionally, there have been instances of persons not known to have polio but now thought to have had a very mild, undiagnosed case of the disease. These individuals may be susceptible to PPS as well. Individuals who do not fit the criteria listed above need to have extensive evaluation before the diagnosis of PPS can be concluded.

Persons at Risk

According to a survey conducted in 1987 by the National Center for Health Statistics, there are more than 1.5 million polio survivors in this country. An estimated 40 percent (approximately six hundred thousand persons) are thought to have had paralytic polio. We now know that even polio survivors who were thought not to have had paralysis may be susceptible to PPS. Unfortunately, these statistics are more than a decade old and are useful only in a very general way.

It is extremely difficult to determine how many polio survivors are alive today in the United States owing to a variety of factors such as poor initial record keeping and a lack of follow-up tracking once the epidemics disappeared. Moreover, sometimes polio survivors are not sure whether they had paralysis or not, for the simple reason that a small child who is feverish and in pain often appears lethargic and even limp. This lack of movement may have been mistakenly interpreted as paralysis when in fact none existed. On the other hand, a child with paralytic polio may wrongly have been thought to be exhausted simply because of a more benign illness and may not have been diagnosed correctly with acute polio.

The estimated number of polio survivors who eventually develop PPS is also controversial and ranges from 25 percent to more than 60 percent. Early studies underestimated the number of polio survivors with PPS probably because many survivors had not yet experienced or complained of new symptoms. More recent studies suggest a much higher proportion. As polio survivors age, it is expected that the majority will experience symptoms related to PPS.

The prognosis for preventing further disability is improving with the availability of exciting new research and medical treatments.

Because developments in the medical field occur daily and often quite unexpectedly, it is crucial that polio survivors maintain a relationship with a medical doctor who specializes in treating polio-related problems including, but not limited to, PPS. There is no substitute for a polio doctor's thoughtful examination in order to assess what might be causing any new ailments and what the best course of treatment might be.

This book is written so that polio survivors and their loved ones can understand more about aging with polio. It is not a replacement for medical treatment. My goal is that it will enable polio survivors to obtain the best medical care available in order to prevent further disability and improve their quality of life as they gracefully age.

CHAPTER 3

Nonparalytic Polio and Post-Polio Syndrome

Throughout history polio has been described in various ways but generally as *paralytic* or *nonparalytic*.[1] Today we are beginning to recognize that there is a spectrum of paralysis, and that individuals who were formerly thought to have had *nonparalytic* polio may have indeed had some mild paralysis. Moreover, recent evidence has suggested that some individuals who were not known to have had polio at all actually did suffer the disease at some point and years later are experiencing symptoms consistent with Post-Polio Syndrome. These cases are anecdotal and in no way reflect the experiences of the majority of polio survivors.

As I was preparing the manuscript for this book, I called Dr. Lauro Halstead and asked him whether he thought nonparalytic polio survivors could have PPS. Not surprisingly, the question had been on his mind as well. He replied that there was almost certainly a spectrum of paralysis, and that individuals not previously thought to have had polio or those who had no weakness when they did have polio may indeed have had unrecognized paralytic polio. In order to explore this issue further, we both reviewed cases we had seen and compared notes. We ended up publishing the first description in the medical literature of nonparalytic polio survivors who were diagnosed with PPS.[2]

The question of whether nonparalytic polio survivors are at risk for PPS is an important one for many reasons. First, a valid diagnosis is essential in order to prescribe appropriate medical treatment. Second, people generally feel reassured when they have an explanation of what is causing their symptoms (particularly when they realize that they do not have a life-threatening condition). Third, a documented diagnosis accepted by the medical community is necessary in order to obtain insurance reimbursement for medical treatment. And fourth, for those individuals who ultimately seek disability benefits, it is imperative to have a diagnosis that is accepted by the medical and scientific communities and is published in the medical literature.

The topic of nonparalytic polio survivors and PPS is still not completely defined. Certainly there are individuals who were not thought to have had paralytic polio who fit the criteria for diagnosis of PPS. Remember that when the polio virus causes illness, individuals generally have a high fever and feel quite sick. It is known that the polio virus invades the gastrointestinal tract *and may go on to invade the nerves in the spinal cord and brain.* Because those who contract polio become quite sick initially, it is common that they go to bed and move very little. It may be difficult to distinguish whether this lack of movement is because they feel generally sick or because they genuinely cannot move well because of mild paralysis. The distinction is particularly difficult to make in children, who (as we have seen) often appear limp and lethargic with any illness causing high fever.

In this chapter I give two examples of individuals who were diagnosed retrospectively with polio. These cases illustrate how confusing it can be to diagnose paralytic polio in retrospect.

A seventy-one-year-old retired surveyor, John Calvin, reported that although he was never diagnosed with polio, he had lived through multiple epidemics in the various towns in which he grew up. In his early twenties, he was discharged from the army and noticed that he was limping on the right side. He went to a Veterans Administration hospital and was given a workup, eventually having corrective surgery to lengthen his right heel cord. He was never given a specific diagnosis; however, it was evident that his right leg was becoming smaller than his left because of muscle atrophy. John functioned fairly well, but in his late sixties he began to have increasing leg weakness on both sides, and profound fatigue. A thorough evaluation was done and John underwent elaborate testing. The conclusion was that at some point in his childhood he had probably contracted polio with very mild paralysis that went unnoticed. Later he developed PPS, which was diagnosed after excluding all other possible causes for his symptoms.

John Calvin was thought to have had polio, but was diagnosed long after the time when he would have had the acute illness. As a young adult, he passed a military physical examination and was able to complete basic training and his other army duties without any problems. As an older adult, however, John began having muscular atrophy in his legs that resulted in significant weakness. It is likely that sometime during his childhood he had an episode where he was sick with a fever and other constitutional symptoms, but was not thought to have paralysis. Therefore, the diagnosis of polio was not made.

In other cases, individuals unambiguously had polio (often because other members of the family had a more severe and noticeable case of paralysis) that was diagnosed at the time of the acute febrile illness, but they were not thought to have paralysis and therefore were mistakenly diagnosed as having nonparalytic polio.

Regardless of whether an initial diagnosis of polio was made, an attempt to establish a history of old polio and to rule out any other medical condition as a cause for new symptoms is critical. In anyone thought to have had the nonparalytic type of polio, the following must be established: (1) that the individual had a likely history of polio, documented by EMG findings consistent with old polio, (2) that the current symptoms fit the diagnostic criteria for PPS, and (3) that other diagnoses have been considered and eliminated. With individuals who were not previously recognized to have had paralytic polio, there is often the problem of trying to establish the initial diagnosis of polio and then considering whether the current symptoms are due to PPS. It is always advisable to get the opinion of a physician who specializes in treating polio survivors, but it is particularly important in persons whose past history of paralytic polio is not well established.

Adding to the confusion is the fact that some individuals were incorrectly diagnosed as having had polio when they actually had an entirely different medical condition. My second example is a woman who was referred to me by her polio support group.

Sandy Bernstein is a forty-five-year-old woman who came to see me because of pain in her knees and increased difficulty in walking. She reported that she had been retrospectively diagnosed as having had "night polio" when she was two years old. At that time her parents had noticed that she was limping and not using her left hand well. Her family doctor told her parents that she had most likely had night polio at some previous time in her short life and that her current problems were a result. Sandy never had any treatment and grew up thinking that she was a polio survivor. When I questioned her further, she primarily complained of problems with coordination rather than true weakness. She also revealed that she had had difficulty in school and had been told by her father that she was "stupid." When I examined

Sandy, I knew immediately that she almost certainly did not have polio, but rather had suffered a stroke either in her mother's womb or shortly after birth. One of the most obvious clues was that she had extremely reactive reflexes on the left side of her body, whereas polio survivors generally have diminished or absent reflexes. When I told Sandy my thoughts, her initial reaction was that I didn't know what I was talking about and she wanted another opinion. I encouraged her to seek a second opinion, but first to get an imaging study of her brain that would positively confirm or deny the presence of an old stroke. Sure enough, Sandy had a lesion on the right side of her brain that was entirely consistent with her history of coordination problems with her left hand and leg, and learning problems in school. The pain in her knees, which I attributed to her abnormal gait pattern, was resolved with physical therapy. Sandy was dumbfounded when I told her the result of the brain scan. She sent her brother, an emergency room physician, a copy of the study results. Although he too was shocked, he confirmed that she did have an old stroke and that this was the root of her problems.

This second example illustrates how easy it is for an individual to be misdiagnosed (particularly when the diagnosis is made long after the original illness is thought to have occurred) and then to carry that diagnosis for a lifetime. Sandy obviously will not get PPS because she never had polio. The treatment I recommended for her is much different from what I would have suggested if she had actually had polio. Although this case represents an error on the part of the family doctor who saw her when she was two years old, other cases of misdiagnosis have occurred when the doctor actually knew or suspected that an individual _did not have polio!_

Because medical insurance was uncommon during the polio epidemics, individuals who contracted polio often had no means of paying what could amount to enormous medical bills. The National

Foundation for Infantile Paralysis (NFIP) was instrumental in raising funds necessary to cover the medical care of nearly all polio survivors in the United States. This fact occasionally led physicians to knowingly misdiagnose individuals who had acute febrile illnesses (but no paralysis) with polio in order to assist them in getting their medical bills covered. These cases are anecdotal, and there is no way to track their frequency. Unfortunately, at this stage it is yet another factor that may cause confusion when trying to confirm an old history of polio in individuals who were diagnosed with nonparalytic polio.

It is becoming increasingly clear that paralytic polio presents as a disease with a wide spectrum of possibilities for weakness—from imperceptible to profound. We now recognize that there are people who were not known to have had polio at all or who were thought to have had a nonparalytic type of polio, who in retrospect almost certainly had a mild case of paralytic polio and today have new medical problems consistent with PPS.

The two examples in this chapter illustrate some of the confusion that surrounds attempts to make the diagnosis of PPS when a history of paralytic polio has never been clearly established. It is important to recognize that some people may not have a classic history of paralytic polio but may indeed have had the disease. Moreover, some of these individuals may be experiencing PPS.

Keep in mind that individuals without a clear history of polio or who were thought to have had nonparalytic polio, who are later recognized to have had a mild case of paralytic polio, are likely to represent a small proportion of the total paralytic polio survivors. Only recently have we recognized these individuals at all. In the future we will undoubtedly know more about how many people are involved and how PPS affects people who have had a very mild (perhaps unrecognizable) case of paralytic polio.

CHAPTER 4

Finding Expert Medical Care

Although nearly every health-care provider in the United States has been involved in one way or another in the care of individuals who have had polio, polio survivors justifiably lament that too often the people who provide this care do not understand their unique medical issues, and in particular do not understand Post-Polio Syndrome. In defense of health-care providers, quite simply, many of them have not had the opportunity to learn about PPS. More often than not, this topic was excluded from their formal didactic training. The key reason is that PPS was not a subject of intense study for scientists and physicians until the 1980s, by which time many of our current health-care providers were already trained.

Frustrated by a lack of resources and knowledgeable medical experts in PPS, polio survivors banded together and formed a network of support groups, newsletters, and (most recently) Internet web sites to share information. The medical world is catching up, though slowly. There are now many excellent rehabilitation centers that specialize in treating polio survivors. These centers are generally located in large cities where academic medical programs exist (see Table 4.1). The doctors who run the clinics often teach at medical

Table 4.1 Resources for finding expert medical care

American Academy of Neurology
1080 Montreal Avenue
St. Paul, MN 55116
http://www.aan.com
(612) 695-1940

American Academy of Orthopedic Surgeons
6300 North River Road
Rosemont, IL 60018-4262
http://www.aaos.org
(847) 823-7186 or (800) 346-AAOS
Fax: (847) 823-8125

American Academy of Physical Medicine and Rehabilitation
One IBM Plaza
Suite 2500
Chicago, IL 60611-3604
http://www.aapmr.org
(312) 464-9700
Fax: (312) 464-0227

Gazette International Networking Institute/International Polio Network
4207 Lindell Boulevard #110
St. Louis, MO 63118-2915
www.post-polio.org
(314) 534-0475

The Polio Society
4200 Wisconsin Avenue, N.W.
Suite 106273
Washington, DC 20016
http://www.polio.org
E-mail: *jshl@mhg.edu*
(301) 897-8180

Note: Reprinted with permission from *Managing Post-Polio.* Courtesy of National Rehabilitation Hospital Press.

schools, participate in research activities, and have a clinical practice in which they treat patients.

The centers that have devoted personnel and resources specifically to treating polio survivors are staffed by a variety of specialists who work together as a team under the leadership of a physician. Most rehabilitation centers with polio programs have one or two physicians in charge of the program and a number of other physicians from different medical specialties who serve as consultants.

Various nonphysician rehabilitation professionals may also participate in the care of polio survivors. These specialists vary according to the polio program, but generally include nurses, occupational and physical therapists, speech and language pathologists, social workers, psychologists, orthotists (brace makers), vocational counselors, and nutritionists. Larger polio programs that cater to out-of-town patients often host clinics that last several days.

While a major rehabilitation center with an established polio program is the ideal place for polio survivors to seek care, it is an option not readily available to some individuals. Consequently, polio survivors may opt to seek care from individual doctors who have expertise in treating the spectrum of polio-related issues. These doctors should ideally be able to refer polio survivors to other specialists in their geographic area when appropriate.

"Polio Doctors"

When looking for medical experts who treat polio-related problems, you will find that the best place to start is with a competent physician. Many individuals have a primary-care physician, either an internist or family practitioner, who oversees most of their medical needs. Most primary-care physicians are not experts in polio-related disease, but ideally will be able to direct polio survivors to another physician in the community who *is* an expert in the field.

Therefore, in addition to their primary-care doctor, whenever possible polio survivors should also choose a "polio doctor," who is most often either a *physiatrist* or a *neurologist*. The polio doctor and the primary-care physician should work together and communicate (generally via letters or office notes) about the care of the individual patient. Both should be integral parts of the continuum of care for polio survivors.

One of the unfortunate aspects of medical cost constraints is that greater emphasis is placed on treatment by primary-care physicians of diseases (ranging from heart disease to cancer) that used to be referred to specialists. Polio survivors should seek care from a specialist if possible, although certainly the primary-care physician should not be ignored. In fact, polio survivors will receive better care overall if the primary-care physician remains informed and involved in their care.

Finding health-care providers who have experience treating polio survivors often hinges on finding a physician who is an expert in polio and the late effects of polio. What follows is a summary of the types of physician experts one can consider consulting.

Physiatrists

Physiatrists are physicians who specialize in Physical Medicine and Rehabilitation (PM&R). The specialty was created in the 1930s and expanded quickly in the 1940s owing in large part to (1) wounded military personnel and (2) the polio epidemics. In the mid-1940s it was obvious that there were not enough trained physiatrists to care for the vast numbers of injured military returnees from World War II. In fact, more than 650,000 wounded military personnel were brought home during that war. According to one historical account, "although 300 Army physicians attended the three-month accelerated course in physiatry under Dr. Krusen at the Mayo Clinic, their numbers were too few to meet the needs of patients."[1]

The need for physicians who understood rehabilitation principles and were able to manage both acute and chronic injuries and illnesses was intensified by the polio epidemics in the first half of the twentieth century. Dr. Robert Bennett, who was chairman of the American Board of PM&R from 1953 to 1963, observed, "I am convinced that it was through contact with patients who had polio that physiatrists first were established as clinicians with the special interest, essential training, and recognized competence to handle those conditions that required carefully prescribed activity."[2]

Because physiatrists were particularly knowledgeable about prescribing exercise therapy for patients, they became known as "the physical therapy doctors." However, physiatrists were physicians who needed to know much more than simply how to prescribe physical therapy. As the specialty evolved, the additional training physiatrists needed after medical school went from three months to four years. In a presidential address to the American Congress of PM&R in 1966, Dr. Lewis Leavitt told his colleagues: "As physicians particularly dedicated to rehabilitation, we have a specific role in the art and practice of medicine today. We are concerned, not exclusively to be sure but in large measure, with the chronic management of physically disabled patients. We must therefore be responsive to the needs and expectations of these patients. Too often in the past, the practice of medicine has largely been limited to diagnosis and treatment of acute illness and disability, with consequent neglect of chronically ill individuals."[3]

Because the polio epidemics helped to shape the medical specialty of PM&R, physiatrists have taken a keen interest in PPS. All physiatrists are trained to treat polio-related issues; in fact, demonstrating competence in treating PPS is integral to passing the medical speciality board examinations in PM&R. However, not all physiatrists are interested in pursuing PPS as a clinical and research interest, so their expertise does not extend beyond the initial training.

The bottom line is that regardless of specialty training, it is highly desirable to find a doctor who has taken a special interest in treating polio survivors. Many physiatrists are excellent polio doctors because of both their early training and their clinical and research interest in all aspects of polio and PPS.

Neurologists

The specialty of modern neurology essentially began after World War I. This growth resulted from the rapidly expanding knowledge of neurologic systems in humans and the development of medical specialties in general. People started to want to go to specialists for a variety of ailments, and physician specialists became increasingly knowledgeable about more specific areas of medicine. The specialty of neurology was a two-way street, with specialists seeking out patients with specific problems and patients seeking out doctors with experience treating those problems. "In addition, specialists initiated assertive and successful advertising campaigns to delineate their distinct services and lure patients to their practices. The growing wealthy class of the industrial revolution provided a focus for these campaigns and willingly supported specialized treatment of their ailments."[4]

Neurology training is similar in duration to the training of physiatrists and also somewhat similar in content. Although there are many differences, with respect to polio and PPS both neurologists and physiatrists are usually taught to manage polio-related issues and to serve as polio doctors. Of course, some neurologists have more interest and expertise than others in polio-related disease; a medical doctor who has the training and interest is ideal.

Further, a good polio doctor can provide the names of other specialists who may be needed to participate in the care of polio survivors. Although neurologists and physiatrists specifically have training in polio and PPS, other doctors with different training backgrounds also make excellent polio doctors. The criterion is a physician who has had extensive experience treating polio survivors and has established a large network of other health-care providers so that all can work together to provide the best possible care.

Orthopedists

The word *orthopaedy* was initially coined in 1741, as the title of a book on the prevention and correction of musculoskeletal disorders by Nicholas Andry, a professor of medicine at the University of Paris. The title was created from two Greek words, *orthos* (straight) and *paidion* (child).[5] Although the term caught on quickly, orthopedics really did not become an organized specialty until the middle to late 1800s. Even so, it took nearly another hundred years before orthopedics reached its current popular status. In fact, in 1941, of the approximately 110,000 physicians in the United States, less than 0.4 percent were certified orthopedic surgeons.[6]

As with physiatrists, the specialty of orthopedic surgery was propelled by both the polio epidemics and the World War II casualties. In the first half of the twentieth century, orthopedists were very concerned with the skeletal deformities that resulted from poliomyelitis. Treatment consisted primarily of exercises, bracing, and surgery. The literature is filled with experimental procedures and surgeries that were being performed for the first time on polio survivors—with mixed success. As the incidence of new cases of polio rapidly declined when the vaccines became widely available, many of the popular orthopedic procedures became almost obsolete.

Modern orthopedists are trained surgeons who are knowledgeable about musculoskeletal conditions that may or may not require surgery. After medical school, orthopedists must complete at least five years of graduate medical education.

Not all orthopedists are familiar with polio-related orthopedic issues. The best way to find an orthopedic surgeon who has experience with polio survivors is to ask a polio doctor or primary-care physician for a referral. Keep in mind that both the primary-care physician and the polio doctor should be consulted about any orthopedic care—especially surgery! Ideally, all physicians involved in a patient's care should at least get copies of office notes and should know what the others are recommending and prescribing.

Physical Therapists

Physical therapy has consistently been a part of the continuum of care for polio and PPS. What many polio survivors are not aware of is how the practice of physical therapy has evolved in the recent past in light of the constraints of the managed-care environment.

Traditionally, when a patient needed physical therapy, his or her doctor would write out a prescription and the patient could choose where to receive the therapy. The patient was evaluated and treated by a registered physical therapist who had at least a four-year college degree (Bachelor of Arts or Science) and often a graduate degree (Master of Science) in physical therapy. Today the facility is often determined by where the patient's health insurance provider has developed a formal contractual relationship. Such facilities may or may not have programs designed for polio survivors. Moreover, the therapists who work there may have little or no experience in treating the late effects of polio.

Another factor is that, in the past, patients routinely worked with a registered physical therapist who cared for them throughout their treatment. As a cost-saving measure in some facilities, a registered physical therapist now does the initial evaluation and then oversees the treatment as the patient works with a physical therapy aide or assistant. The main difference between working with an aide or assistant and working with a registered physical therapist is the level of formal education. A physical therapy aide may have no formal training at all, whereas a physical therapy assistant has completed a two-year program of study and has an associate's degree. On the other hand, these titles represent formal training in school only, and do not provide information about the therapist's experience. Some physical therapy assistants and even aides may have excellent skills in working with polio survivors. Once again, the best way to find an appropriate therapist is to ask a polio doctor for the name of someone skilled in treating polio survivors.

Physical therapists play a critical role in the treatment of polio-related issues including PPS. In general, they are expert at prescribing appropriate exercises, can help treat and sometimes cure painful musculoskeletal conditions, and can prescribe and instruct on the use of various assistive devices (canes, crutches, and the like), shoe orthotics, and braces. Physical therapists are also experts at improving home and work environments to make them safer and easier for persons with disabilities. Often they will perform an on-site evaluation. Physical therapists can be resources for a variety of other types of information that may depend on their personal expertise and experience.

Occupational Therapists

Occupational therapists also play a critical role in rehabilitation settings. As with physical therapy, there is a three-tiered hierarchy, with occupational therapists having the most formal education. Next in line are occupational therapy assistants, followed by occupational therapy aides. Of course, the amount of formal education does not always predict who will do the most competent job. A good polio doctor will be able to advise you in this regard.

The role of the occupational therapist is to focus on how people accomplish what they need to do each day, whether it be bathing and dressing, traveling, household chores, or working outside the home. In rehabilitation terms, these are referred to as activities of daily living, or ADLs for short. The occupational therapist's job is to teach people the skills they require to do the things they need to do each day. Often special equipment, termed *adaptive equipment,* is used. For instance, if someone has difficulty bending over, they may be shown how to use a long shoehorn. Or if a person has difficulty reaching overhead items, she or he may learn to use a device called a reacher.

Occupational therapists are also experts in treating arm and hand injuries. In this respect they may have a significant crossover of skills with physical therapists, who also may be quite skilled at treating upper-extremity injuries such as tendinitis or frozen shoulder. In my own polio clinic, the occupational therapists are also responsible for teaching polio survivors how to pace themselves. This instruction is tailored to each person's lifestyle and needs. Each participant in the clinic is asked to fill out a three-day log of activities (see Chapter 14), which is designed to help the occupational therapist in assessing a polio survivor who may need to utilize some pacing techniques for energy conservation.

The occupational therapist should also work with the physical therapist to review if and when someone is falling or tripping. Since falls often result in significant further disability, therapists should be acutely attentive to trying to limit such occurrences. Depending on the setup of the clinic, either the occupational or physical therapist or both may have this responsibility. Although there is some overlap between the two, their roles in any particular polio clinic are usually quite well defined. Furthermore, both occupational and physical therapists work closely with the physician in charge as well as with other health-care professionals in order to provide comprehensive care for polio survivors.

Many other health-care providers play an integral role in the rehabilitation setting. These experts may include orthotists (brace makers), social workers, psychologists, vocational rehabilitation counselors, recreational therapists, nurses, and nutritionists. Depending on the geographic location, size of the polio clinic, and structure of the polio program, several or all of these specialists may be available for consultation.

Trying to find specialists in the treatment of polio-related disease may seem overwhelming. Remember that it is best to start with a doctor who is an expert in managing the medical issues unique to polio survivors. Physicians who are truly expert in treating polio survivors will have a large network of colleagues in a variety of medical specialties. The ability to refer polio survivors to appropriate health-care professionals is an integral part of a polio doctor's expertise. Moreover, since physicians direct and supervise the care of their patients and write orders for therapists and other health-care providers, they need to be intimately aware of where their patients are being treated. Thus, finding a polio doctor is a crucial first step in managing all polio-related medical issues—including PPS.

CHAPTER 5

The EMG Controversy

Polio survivors who are seeking medical treatment are often faced with the dilemma of whether or not to have an electromyographic study (EMG). The decision to proceed or decline should be carefully considered and based on accurate information regarding what the study entails and what information is garnered from it.

An EMG is a *physiological* test that studies how the muscles are working. The fact that it actually tests what is occurring at the level of the muscles—as opposed to *imaging* tests (essentially high-tech photographs) such as magnetic resonance imaging studies (MRIs), bone scans, computed tomography scans (CTs), and the like—means that the information it provides is different from that provided by other studies. This unique quality of the EMG makes it a valuable tool in some instances. The actual test involves placing a fine sterile needle into the muscles and measuring their actions on a screen. The needle is moved from place to place, so that different muscles are tested. No electrical impulses are used. One can think of the needle as a small television camera that records what the muscles are doing. The EMG is capable of determining whether there has been an injury to the muscles being tested, what might have caused the injury, and whether the injury is old or new.

Table 5.1 Comparison of EMG and NCS

Electromyography (EMG):	Nerve Conduction Studies (NCS):
Uses a sterile, disposable needle that is inserted into the muscle	Use electrodes that adhere to the skin (but do not penetrate)
No electrical impulses are used	Involve small electrical impulses (shocks)
Measures what is happening to the muscles (which the nerves supply)	Measure how the nerves are working

The EMG is generally combined with another study called a nerve conduction study (NCS). This test involves using surface electrodes (no needles) that are applied painlessly to the skin. A small stimulator held by the person performing the study is placed near the electrodes and electrical impulses (shocks) are administered. These electrical impulses test how fast and how well the nerves are able to respond. Thus, the NCS differs from the EMG in that it does not involve a needle, but rather uses small electrical impulses. The NCS is also different in that it *directly tests the nerves,* whereas the EMG *directly studies the muscles* and *indirectly gathers information about the nerves.* Both studies involve some discomfort, although most people find them quite tolerable, particularly when the individual performing the test is skilled (see Table 5.1).

Both the EMG and the NCS are often recommended for polio survivors in order to evaluate injury to the nerves and muscles from the initial polio, and to determine whether any new muscle or nerve problems are occurring. The tests complement each other in that each provides information that may be vital in order to treat nerve and muscle conditions. Furthermore, this information may not be obtainable in any other way. Information from the EMG and NCS may be interpreted using information from other tests as well. It is rather like putting together the pieces of a puzzle: the picture only becomes clear when all of the pieces are joined. The other tests most often recommended are blood tests and imaging studies.

In order to understand how these tests work together (and why one of them alone may not be sufficient) think of the doctor who recommends them as a chef who needs milk, flour, butter, and eggs. The combination of these ingredients can make a delectable pastry. Any one ingredient alone, while edible, does not have the same taste. A skilled physician is able to order a variety of tests that in combination are able to definitively diagnose different medical conditions. Any one of the tests alone may not provide enough information to make a correct diagnosis.

The EMG (and NCS) in Polio Survivors

There are two primary reasons why EMG and NCS studies are controversial in polio survivors: first, because the tests are often uncomfortable, and second, because they are expensive. If the tests were painless and free, it is likely that there would be no controversy and most polio survivors experiencing new symptoms would undergo both studies. However, the reality is that these studies are not painless or free, so the question of whether to have these tests done needs to be addressed.

There are two main reasons to have an EMG and NCS. First, these studies help to identify whether an individual had polio in the past and to what extent the arms and legs were involved. *These studies do not absolutely confirm a history of old polio, but help to corroborate patients' recollections.* Consequently, EMG and NCS studies are an integral part of the accepted diagnostic criteria for PPS, as discussed in Chapter 2. Many times individuals are not entirely certain whether they had polio, so these studies can help to determine what type of injury, if any, occurred to their nerves and muscles. Other individuals may have been told they had polio but were misdiagnosed. The new studies may help establish the correct diagnosis. Even if there is no question about previous polio, these studies can be helpful in determining the extent of muscle involvement.

Physicians who are experts in treating polio survivors are able to interpret the results of the NCS and EMG studies and make recommendations based on what has been found. For instance, an individual who has EMG evidence of old polio in his arms and legs and presents with new weakness involving all the limbs might be prescribed a different exercise program than someone who has EMG evidence of old polio only in the legs and is experiencing new weakness there. One might argue that the exercise program could be prescribed based on the individual's history and physical examination; however, consider for a moment the second case, in which the individual's arms do not reveal any evidence of old polio. What if the EMG *had* revealed signs of old polio? Would the prescribed exercise program be different? Many polio experts would say yes. If the arms are not involved, a more vigorous arm exercise program is often prescribed, whereas if testing reveals that the arms are involved (even if the individual is not currently complaining of arm weakness) a less vigorous arm exercise program is likely. Remember that in an individual who has had polio and has lost some of the nerves that supply the muscles in the arms, an overly aggressive exercise program may cause permanent arm weakness.

The second reason why someone might want to have NCS and EMG studies performed is that they are very effective in picking up other nerve and muscle problems not related to the initial polio but frequently encountered in polio survivors. In one study, nearly 50 percent of polio survivors studied had evidence of other nerve problems that were treatable and often curable.[1] Untreated, these problems can potentially lead to significant weakness in the arms and legs, causing further disability as well as pain and suffering. The next question might be, Why doesn't everyone have these studies done as screening tests, in the way mammograms are recommended for women? The answer is that these studies are considerably more useful in people who have had polio because these individuals are much more likely to have additional nerve and muscle problems. Polio survivors have a high risk for new nerve and muscle injuries for a variety of reasons that include the inadequately supported skeletal structures (due to the initial paralysis), overuse of the arms and legs, and direct pressure on nerves that are not sufficiently protected by other tissues. Consequently, polio survivors are much more likely to have new nerve injuries that can easily be detected by EMG and NCS.

The importance of obtaining objective data in order to confirm a diagnosis cannot be overstated. Often polio survivors need this information in order to justify to insurance companies why certain services should be covered. As the health-care system is in a state of flux and insurers are looking for ways to cut spending, one of the first items to be erased is benefits for "chronic" conditions such as polio and PPS. A new diagnosis such as carpal tunnel syndrome (median neuropathy), which legitimately requires medical attention and possibly more services from home-care providers, is essential to document. If a new problem exists, objective tests such as an EMG and NCS are very sensitive and specific for different types of nerve and muscle conditions, and they are well-respected studies in the medical community.

We have seen that despite the discomfort and the cost, there are compelling reasons why individuals who have had polio may want to undergo EMG and NCS; nevertheless, there are circumstances in which a polio survivor might want to forgo testing—for instance, if the test is deemed too painful or too costly. If the treating physician is not inclined to order the test because of low suspicion of any new problems and he or she is confident about the diagnosis of previous polio, then the study may not be very useful. A physician who is a polio expert should be able to appropriately recommend if and when NCS and EMG studies should be undertaken.

CHAPTER 6

Prevailing over Pain

There is an oft-told saying that the only things one can count on in life are death and taxes. Pain should be added to this list, for everyone suffers pain. In fact, a recurrent theme from birth to death is pain and the suffering that accompanies it. Clearly for some individuals pain's grip is more enduring, more severe, more disabling than for others. Most polio survivors are intimately familiar with pain from the time of onset of the acute illness, if not before.

Pain mixed with feelings of helplessness and uncertainty about the future is well documented by survivors who have written their memoirs. The noted children's author Peg Kehret describes a nurse's response to her request for help when she was in pain: " 'I am too busy to run in here just to turn you in that bed.' She shook a finger at me. 'Don't you call me again unless it's an emergency. You hear me? Do not call me unless you can't breathe.' My legs throbbed, my arms ached, my back, neck, and throat hurt. I lay there, helpless, staring at her. She could have turned me in the time it took to tell me no, I thought."[1]

Fortunately, once the acute febrile illness subsides, so does the pain. For most polio survivors pain is not a prominent feature in their lives until decades later when they begin experiencing pain that often is severe and disabling. Studies have indicated that the majority of polio survivors have pain—regardless of whether they have been diagnosed with Post-Polio Syndrome. Frequently the pain occurs on a daily basis and affects the quality of life.

In order to better understand pain and its influence on any given medical condition, consider the following:

1. Pain is a symptom and is not itself a medical condition.
2. Pain is a result of chemical messages in the brain and is really the mechanism by which the body lets the brain know that something is wrong.
3. Nearly any medical condition that alters one's body from its usual state may result in pain as a symptom.
4. Pain can be a symptom of a very serious or of a relatively inconsequential medical condition.
5. The severity of the pain does not necessarily correlate with the severity of the underlying medical condition (mild pain may be the first sign of a serious medical condition, or severe pain may be associated with a medical condition that is minor and easily treated).

Since pain is a message from the brain, it is useful to think of pain as your body's communicating this announcement: "Something is wrong—go to your doctor to find out what it is and how it should be treated." Unfortunately, some people hear the pain message as "Something is wrong—if you ignore it long enough, it might go away." Or they hear: "Something is wrong—be stalwart and endure without complaining or seeking help."

I am not suggesting that people rush to their doctors for every bruise or scrape, *but rather for any pain that is undiagnosed and/or has been present for more than two weeks.* Many painful conditions, regardless of how serious they are, will not go away without appropriate treatment. If something fails to disappear on its own, you need to find out what it is, particularly in the event that it may become disabling or even life threatening.

It is vital to keep in mind that *any pain, regardless of its origin, can contribute to further disability.* It has been learned that pain negatively influences polio survivors in a number of ways, including energy level, mobility, sleep, and emotions.[2]

Intuitively it makes sense that if individuals are experiencing pain, they will not feel like doing, and may not be able to do, the activities they normally enjoy. They may feel sad and frustrated, particularly if they also are not sleeping well at night owing to the pain. Scientific studies have documented this vicious cycle of having pain, doing less, sleeping poorly, and feeling depressed. Even if the origin of the pain is a rather simple treatable condition such as tendinitis, this cycle can develop and can become *disabling*. Thus, all painful conditions that last more than two weeks should be evaluated by a medical doctor who can then prescribe appropriate treatment.

Acute versus Chronic Pain

Pain is frequently classified as *acute* or *chronic*. The two differ only in the length of time they have been present. Acute pain has been present for days to weeks, chronic pain for months to years. With chronically painful conditions, an individual may have only had pain intermittently but it has recurred over a long period.

The treatment of acute and chronic pain may differ significantly depending on what is causing the pain and what treatment has been rendered in the past. A rule of thumb is that the longer the pain has been present, the more difficult it is to treat. This is particularly true if many treatment options have been tried unsuccessfully. On the other hand, persons with a chronic painful condition that has not been diagnosed or has been misdiagnosed have a much better chance of seeing improvement in their symptoms once the correct diagnosis is made and proper treatment is given. No matter what is causing the pain or how long the pain has been present, keep in mind that help, and usually substantial relief, are available for most painful medical conditions that are accurately diagnosed and appropriately treated.

Pain in Polio Survivors

Pain in polio survivors can be further classified into three types.[3] Type I pain, described as post-polio muscle pain (PPMP), frequently occurs as a superficial burning or a deep muscle ache. Type II pain occurs because of injury to soft tissues such as the tendons, ligaments, and muscles. Examples include tendinitis, bursitis, muscle strains, and ligament sprains. Type III pain, described as *biomechanical pain*, is the result of arthritis that occurs with aging, low back pain due to weakness and poor lumbar support, and so on. Nerve injuries to the spine or extremities are also classified as Type III pain.

This classification system is useful for musculoskeletal conditions only. Many other medical illnesses may cause pain that does not fit into any of these categories (stomach ulcer, cancer, heart disease causing angina, and so forth). Fortunately, the most common painful conditions in polio survivors are related to one of the three types listed above (none of which are life threatening); however, it is always important to seek out a physician's medical diagnosis of any painful condition.

Only Type I pain is reviewed in detail here. The diagnoses associated with Types II and III are beyond the scope of this chapter.

Post-polio muscle pain typically occurs in the muscles (rather than the joints or other areas of the body) and is often described as a burning, cramping, aching, or "tired" feeling. It is *not* described as a sharp shooting pain associated with tingling or electrical feelings, which often signify a nerve injury. PPMP, very common in polio survivors, is associated with muscular use and, most probably, *overuse*. Thus, polio experts advise survivors that if they pace themselves and avoid overusing their muscles, they will generally experience less muscular aching and cramping.

The obvious question is, How much is too much? That is to say, When are polio survivors overusing their muscles? In order to answer this question, think back for a moment to the earlier definition of pain as a symptom of a medical condition. The medical condition is Post-Polio Syndrome, and the symptom of PPMP is thought to occur because of muscular strain and fatigue. Therefore, the best way to determine whether individuals are overusing their muscles is to have them monitor their muscular pain symptoms. If people are experiencing a lot of PPMP, chances are that they are overusing their muscles and need to decrease their activity level. Obviously, the only people who can do this are those who are in touch with their bodies and are willing to modify their activity level based on how much pain they are experiencing.

Classically, PPMP occurs at night and tends to be worse when an individual has had a very active day, yet many polio survivors find that their PPMP does not fit this scenario. I often hear individuals lament that they are unable to correlate their pain level with their activity level. Although many who pace themselves and take frequent rest periods are able to manage their muscle pain easily, others are not so fortunate. Some polio survivors have PPMP throughout the day or experience it more in the morning, regardless of their activity level. Whether someone has "classic" PPMP or not, a thoughtful history and physical examination are in order in case there are unidentified sources of the pain.

If an individual has been diagnosed with PPMP and it is not controlled with activity modification, other treatment options are available. Since different treatments work in different people, it is impossible to generalize and predict the best method to control PPMP. The topic of medications warrants further discussion, as do complementary and alternative medicine (massage, acupuncture, magnets), often used to treat painful conditions. These treatments are discussed briefly in this chapter and in more detail in Chapter 22.

Medications to Treat or Control Pain

Medications used in the treatment of pain fall into different categories. The most common are anti-inflammatory medications (often called NSAIDS), antidepressant medications, antiseizure medications, and narcotic medications. Other drugs used do not fit into these categories; however, those listed are the most commonly prescribed.

Anti-inflammatory medications, which work to treat pain and inflammation, are called by a number of different names (ibuprofen, naproxen, piroxicam). Despite some subtle differences, they work more or less in the same manner. Their major side effect is irritation of the stomach lining, which may result in bleeding or an ulcer— very serious and potentially life threatening. Fortunately, for individuals who are unable to tolerate the traditional anti-inflammatory medications, some newer ones have far fewer reports of gastrointestinal side effects, such as heartburn or ulcers.

When taking anti-inflammatory medications, people often mistakenly assume that they are just "pain killers" and fail to take them as prescribed. Since a consistent blood level is needed to attack inflammation, taking them only occasionally may limit their ability to treat the inflammatory aspect of a medical condition—which is a critical part of the healing process.

Antidepressant medications are used in a variety of ways to help control pain. Although several subclasses are beyond the scope of this chapter, in general they work by changing some of the chemical signals in the brain in order to alleviate pain. They may also improve one's mood and help with sleep. (As noted above, chronic pain can result in poor sleep and an unpleasant mood—both of which feed into the cycle of continued chronic pain.) In polio survivors, the class known as tricyclic antidepressant medications has been noted to help with PPMP.

Antiseizure medications change the chemicals in the nervous system in order to help relax the muscles and stabilize the nerve membranes (making them less irritable and painful).

As noted above, a variety of different medications can be used to treat pain. The first and most important consideration is to determine what is being treated—that is, what is the diagnosis? An answer will significantly narrow the choices, and then the decision will be which medication is most likely to be effective and least likely to cause intolerable side effects? Keep in mind that all medications have potential side effects!

Complementary and Alternative Medicine to Manage Pain

When it comes to anything other than medications and physical or occupational therapy (both of which need to be carefully prescribed by a polio doctor familiar with PPMP), my philosophy is that individuals who are experiencing pain (and have checked with their doctors) can try alternative medical treatments as long as the treatments do not harm them and are not exorbitantly expensive or time-consuming. My one caveat is that I routinely advise polio survivors to avoid most manipulation procedures (chiropractic manipulation or forceful manipulation with massage, physical or occupational therapy), because of the possibility of injury. Although widely practiced, these manipulative techniques have serious potential complications such as spinal cord injury with resultant paralysis, fractures, nerve injuries, and so forth. Particularly for polio survivors who have weakness and decreased bone density, the possibility of injury from a manipulative procedure is an unnecessary risk.

Ten Steps to Improving PPMP

1. Have a doctor evaluate the pain, to be certain that it is truly PPMP and not pain from a different etiology. Follow through on the physician's recommendations for further testing and treatment.

2. Keep a pain and activity diary to try and determine if and how the PPMP is affected by activity (see Chapter 14 for an example of a three-day log).

3. Try to modify your activities and see whether you notice a difference in your pain level. Decreasing physical stress and strain can often improve symptoms of PPMP. You may want to expand or repeat the three-day log after modifying your activities, to see if this has any effect on your pain level.

4. Take an inventory of your current mobility status. Keep in mind that mobility, regardless of the method, takes an enormous toll on your muscles. Do you need to get new braces or have your old ones repaired? Should you consider using a cane? Would it help to use a motorized scooter or wheelchair, even if part-time? (Refer to Chapters 18–20 for more on mobility, bracing, and scooters and wheelchairs.) If your doctor has not already recommended that you see a physical therapist for a mobility evaluation, consider asking if this would be beneficial.

If modifying your activities is not enough to manage the PPMP (or if for some reason you are unable to modify your activities to the level where your pain is controlled), then consider the following additional steps:

5. Consult a doctor for recommendations on medications that may be helpful in controlling PPMP.

6. Try formal physical or occupational therapy to decrease symptoms of PPMP through gentle strengthening and stretching exercises. Gentle massage may also be helpful, as can improving posture and balance. In addition, physical and occupational therapists

are skilled in using modalities such as ultrasound, heat, ice, and electrical stimulation in order to decrease pain symptoms.

7. Ask about muscular injections, for instance trigger-point injections used to decrease pain if the muscles in spasm are confined to a specific area. These injections are ineffective for muscle aches that occur throughout the arms and legs, but may be useful for neck pain, upper-arm or leg pain, and the like.

8. Seek recommendations about specialized equipment designed to reduce muscular stress and strain. Generally called adaptive equipment, it may be anything from a shower seat to a long-handled shoehorn. Occupational and physical therapists can suggest adaptive equipment to reduce muscular overuse.

9. Consider complementary and alternative medicine (CAM); these treatments are discussed in Chapter 22.

10. Try to improve your sleep, stress level, and mood. All pain is worse in individuals who are not sleeping well and/or are under severe emotional stress. Pain symptoms are also exacerbated by feelings of isolation and depression (understandably this often creates a vicious cycle, for someone's feelings of depression would not be as prominent if the person experienced less pain and vice versa).

CHAPTER 7

Preserving and Protecting Your Arms

Every polio survivor whom I have had the pleasure of treating has heard me say at least once, "Your arms are your key to independence." Think about it. If you cannot use your legs at all, you can still remain totally independent—living alone, bathing yourself, feeding yourself, driving a car. But if you cannot use your *arms* at all, you immediately cease to be independent and must rely on others to help you with even the most routine (and intimate) activities of daily living. For polio survivors who are completely self-sufficient, the thought of relinquishing even a small amount of their independence is distressing. Others who have had arm paralysis since their acute illness, and have relied on caregivers for assistance, fear that further injury to their arms would render them even more disabled. Because the arms are absolutely critical in order to function as independently as possible, I am devoting an entire chapter to preserving strength and preventing injuries in the upper extremities.

As a start, it is imperative to understand what might potentially affect a polio survivor's arm function. Although there are many medical conditions that may adversely affect the arms, for the sake of consistency I will present them in the same manner as in Chapter 6.

The redundancy in the two chapters is unavoidable; however, the topics presented are important enough to justify the repetition.

Type I: Post-Polio Muscle Pain

Post-polio muscle pain (PPMP) typically occurs in the muscles rather than in the joints; pain localized to the shoulder, elbow, wrist, or fingers is most likely not PPMP. Often described as aching, cramping, burning, or a "tired" feeling, PPMP frequently occurs at night or after the polio survivor has been very active. As the neglected workhorses of the upper body, the arms are particularly susceptible to PPMP. Any warning of overuse of the muscles should be heeded, and the arms should be rested as much as possible. The best way to combat PPMP is steadfastly to avoid overuse and stress of the arm muscles. (Other treatment options are discussed in detail in Chapter 6.) The diagnosis of PPMP may be elusive, since it may occur in the arms even if they were not thought to be involved at the time of the initial polio. A careful evaluation is vital with any upper-extremity pain.

Although many polio survivors intermittently experience PPMP, one must be exceedingly careful not to immediately reach the conclusion that whatever arm pain they are experiencing is PPMP. For PPMP can occur in polio survivors whether or not they have Post-Polio Syndrome. However, PPMP is one of the symptoms of PPS and is diagnosed *after excluding all other potential causes of arm pain.* Erroneously assuming that the pain in question is due to PPMP while another underlying (potentially treatable or curable) medical condition goes undiagnosed may lead to disastrous results and permanent disability in the arms.

Juanita Carlos is a petite forty-five-year-old woman who came from out of state for a one-time consultation with me. Although she had paralytic polio as a child, Juanita's recovery was remarkable. One would have to look closely to see any evidence that polio was once a part of her life. Despite how well she looked, Juanita was experiencing increasing symptoms of pain, weakness, numbness, and tingling in her hands. Told that she had PPS, she was convinced that she was doomed to a fate of progressive disability. When she unexpectedly called me, I explained that her symptoms were not entirely consistent with PPMP and that she needed a careful evaluation of her upper extremities. Juanita gathered up her medical records and came to see me for the sole purpose of trying to figure out what was causing her symptoms and how best to keep her arms functional. What I found surprised me.

On two separate occasions, Juanita had had nerve conduction studies documenting nerve injuries in her arms. The second study looked worse than the first, signifying that the injuries were becoming more severe. Her physical examination was equally disturbing. She had marked atrophy of the muscles of her hands, with profound weakness and loss of sensation. When I explained to Juanita that the weakness and sensory loss in her hands was almost certainly caused by the nerve injury, she was dismayed. Her doctor had explained that she had some nerve injury, but she did not regard it as a serious problem. Sadly, Juanita told me they had never discussed treatment options or prognosis. Because her doctor had said he was "following" the nerve injuries via the nerve conduction studies, Juanita assumed that nothing more could be done. When she became increasingly disabled, Juanita believed the cause was PPMP and that she should simply rest her arms as much as possible.

Juanita's story has haunted me as I have continued to counsel polio survivors. So much could have been done before she got to the point where she was unable to tie her shoes, button her buttons, or type on her computer. At the time of the first nerve conduction study, I would have considered recommending splints for her wrists, elbow pads, oral medications, occupational or physical therapy, and possibly injections to help heal the injured nerves. If these measures had been unsuccessful, after the second study I would likely have recommended surgical release of the compressed nerves. Early treatment would have stopped the progression of the weakness and sensory loss, and Juanita might even have regained some of her lost strength and sensation. As it was, all I could do was tell her that surgery was her best option in order to prevent still further weakness and sensory loss. In all likelihood, because the nerves had been compressed for such a long period, surgery would not restore any of her former function.

This is an example of the disastrous results that can occur when polio survivors erroneously assume (or are told) that their symptoms are due to PPMP. Once again, *for anyone experiencing symptoms in their arms, there is no substitute for a meticulous examination by a doctor who specializes in treating polio survivors.*

Type II: Soft-Tissue Injuries

For the purposes of this discussion, soft-tissue injuries are those that affect the muscles, tendons, and ligaments of the arms. They are generally classified as muscle strains, ligament sprains, tendinitis, or bursitis. Although Type II injuries may also be due to overuse, they typically are self-limited injuries that can affect multiple structures and may involve inflammation. Often these injuries occur in the arms from repetitive activities such as using a computer, chopping vegetables, playing a musical instrument, knitting, or woodworking. Such injuries are classified by a variety of names, all of which mean essentially the same thing: repetitive motion injuries, repetitive strain injuries, or cumulative trauma disorders. In polio survivors, these types of soft-tissue injuries occur frequently and often without an obvious reason. This is because many polio survivors have some upper-body weakness (which may be subtle) that makes their arms more susceptible to injury. Also, polio survivors who have decreased lower-body strength tend to rely on their arms to assist them with mobility (as in getting up from a chair or making a transfer). This, too, may increase the susceptibility of the arms to injury.

Nearly always, soft-tissue injuries present with pain that may only be noticeable during specific arm maneuvers. Most of these injuries are treatable and often curable, so an early and accurate diagnosis by a medical doctor is essential. Ignoring arm pain, new weakness, or loss of range of motion in the joints is hazardous to one's health and future function. A "minor" upper-extremity injury may turn into a chronic condition or may become a "major" upper-extremity injury—both of which lead directly to further disability.

As an example, consider the tendons of the shoulder. This group of tendons, commonly referred to as the rotator cuff, helps to stabilize the shoulder joint, particularly when the arm is lifted overhead. These tendons can develop a tendinitis (inflammation) that is usually quite easily treated with medications, icing, and sometimes physical therapy. If the tendinitis is present for months or years without appropriate treatment, the tendons may weaken and tear. A tear of the rotator cuff (particularly a complete tear of the tendons involved) is much more serious than a simple tendinitis. Rotator cuff tears may result in inability to lift the arm overhead and often require surgery in an attempt to reattach the tendons. Rotator cuff tears can occur at any time, but an underlying untreated tendinitis of extended duration may increase the likelihood.

Treatment for soft-tissue injuries of the upper extremities depends on the diagnosis, the severity of the symptoms, and where in the arms they are located. The many possibilities are usually quite effective: avoidance of activities that exacerbate the symptoms, ice, heat, splints, oral medications, injections, physical and occupational therapy, and (in rare instances) surgery. Keep in mind that these treatment options and others work only when an appropriate initial diagnosis has been made. Self-diagnosis and treatment are to be avoided. They are not likely to help and may even make the condition worse.

Type III: Biomechanical Pain

Biomechanical pain includes age-related changes due to arthritis, muscle weakness leading to poor trunk support, and nerve injuries in the spine and extremities. Type III pain generally presents as neck pain and joint pain. If a nerve injury occurs, it may present as a tingling pain sometimes associated with numbness and weakness of the arms. Most people, regardless of whether they have had polio, intermittently experience biomechanical pain—particularly as they age. For polio survivors, biomechanical pain is often much more prominent than in others owing to weakness that prevents adequate support of the body's skeletal structure. As with all pain issues described in this chapter, a polio doctor who is familiar with the complexities and nuances of biomechanical pain in polio survivors is the best person to make an assessment.

Often biomechanical pain is attributed to "arthritis" and is thought to be untreatable. But even if arthritis is present, it may not be the major source of the pain. An example is the often-overlooked and misdiagnosed neck-pain syndrome that results in headaches at the back of the head. The neck pain is commonly called a cervical myofascial pain syndrome, and the headache is called a suboccipital neuralgia (Figure 7.1). Both the neck pain and the headaches are due to muscle spasm and strain rather than to arthritis. Even if arthritis is present, it can usually be successfully treated because the major source of pain is the muscles around the neck rather than the joints in the spine.

I give this example because I have found that a lot of polio

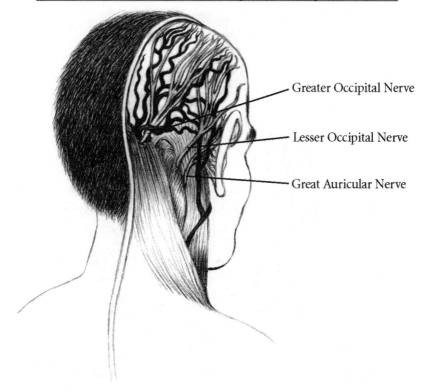

Greater Occipital Nerve

Lesser Occipital Nerve

Great Auricular Nerve

Fig. 7.1. Muscles around the neck and the back of the head can tighten around nerves, causing pain and headaches. This is called occipital neuralgia.

survivors have neck pain and headaches—sometimes severe and disabling—in the backs of their heads. Part of the reason is upper-body weakness that may result in poor posture and muscular strain. Fortunately, these injuries usually resolve when correctly diagnosed and treated.

Initial treatment may include improving one's sitting posture and avoiding neck strain, physical therapy, massage, heat, oral medications, and topical creams. If these treatments fail, injections may be useful. Two types of injections may help: the first is trigger-point

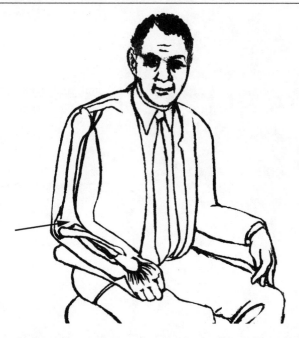

Fig. 7.2. The ulnar nerve (arrow) is very superficial and therefore vulnerable at the inside (medial side) of the elbow. Pressure on the elbow may cause injury to the nerve, leading to loss of sensation and weakness. The left-hand figure demonstrates the incorrect way to position elbows. The right-hand figure demonstrates how forearm rests (or data arms) can support the arms distal to the elbow, so the ulnar nerve is protected.

injections into the muscles below the level of the nerves, which may help the muscles to relax and loosen their grip on the nerves; the second is an actual nerve block that involves placing medication at the level of the nerves and blocking the pain that stems from this level. Injections tend to be very effective for this type of problem if all else fails.

Finally, nerve injuries are another source of pain that is too often overlooked, misdiagnosed, or simply not taken seriously enough. *It is absolutely critical to diagnose and treat nerve injuries early because*

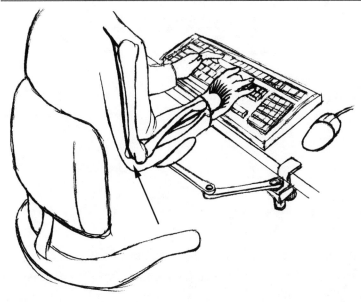

they often lead to further weakness that may be permanent. Studies reveal that polio survivors are susceptible to nerve injuries in their arms because of multiple factors, including the use of crutches and canes, and poor arm positioning in chairs and wheelchairs. These injuries may be improved or avoided altogether by understanding the basic anatomy and avoiding pressure on the part of the arm where the nerve is most vulnerable (Figure 7.2). Surgery for nerve injuries is often an option, but many of these injuries can be treated and potentially cured without surgery if they are caught early. If numbness and tingling are present, they are not symptoms associated with Type I or Type II pain; one should be extremely suspicious of a nerve injury.

CHAPTER 8

Sustaining Strength

Probably the greatest fear of polio survivors is that they will become weaker with time. After the enormous effort made to regain strength following the initial polio bout, the thought of once again becoming weak seems incomprehensible. Nevertheless, many polio survivors are facing what they fear most—increased weakness. Regrettably, in many individuals this new weakness is directly linked to further disability. Although new weakness is one of the cardinal signs of Post-Polio Syndrome, many factors may contribute to a loss of strength in polio survivors.

Studies have shown that everyone loses some strength as they age.[1] However, polio survivors appear to lose strength faster than the norm.[2] Additionally, they often describe new weakness in limbs not previously thought to have been affected by the initial polio. How and why this occurs is the subject of many debates. Although there are numerous theories, the new weakness probably is due to several factors that together have a more marked effect than any one alone would. The most important of these factors are the following:

Normal aging
Lack of reserve strength
Overuse of the muscles

Disuse of the muscles
Other medical conditions

It is known that aging individuals lose strength over time. This "normal" loss of strength is now considered to be less significant than was thought in the past. Recent studies have indicated that the combined effects of a sedentary lifestyle (disuse of the muscles) and other medical conditions (such as heart disease or diabetes) act synergistically to accelerate what was once considered normal aging of the muscles.[3] In polio survivors, two other factors tend to accelerate (or give the appearance of accelerating) this process still more. The first is overuse of the muscles, which most likely does contribute to accelerated aging; the second is the absence of the reserve strength that was lost during the initial bout with polio, which often gives the *appearance* of accelerated aging.

In order to understand how overuse of some muscles and disuse of others may unwittingly occur, consider the following.

At one talk I gave to polio survivors, a woman was present who remained unconvinced that she was doing more harm than good by using a manual (rather than a motorized) wheelchair. "But this is how I keep my arms strong!" she exclaimed. More than once I have heard polio survivors say that using a manual wheelchair is an excellent form of exercise for their arms. But I firmly disagree. Using a manual wheelchair involves the same motions over and over. Some muscles do a lot of work while others are not much involved. Moreover, the amount of work done by propelling the wheelchair is inconsistent on any given day. All of us move more on some days than on other days. Wheelchair propulsion as a means of exercising the upper extremities makes no sense in light of the risk of overuse of some muscles and disuse of others. Moreover, all forms of exercise (particularly in polio survivors) should have consistent parameters (the amount of time performed, the amount of resistance, the number of repetitions). The inherent variability of what a given individual needs to accomplish on a particular day (thereby propelling the wheelchair either more or less) means that the parameters for this "exercise" are not consistent and may lead to overuse and even permanent weakness. Often individuals substitute for exercise daily activities (such as propelling a wheelchair or going up and down stairs) that may cause muscular overuse and further weakness, instead of establishing a formal and controlled exercise program designed to build strength and improve fitness.

A loss of reserve strength from the initial polio illness is a confounding variable in how polio survivors' strength is maintained as they age. Here is an example I often use.

A certain threshold of strength is needed to do any given activity. Imagine that it takes 30 percent of your total arm strength to lift a gallon of milk. This means that 30 percent is the threshold of strength your arm needs to be able to lift the milk; if your strength falls below that mark, you are unable to lift the milk. If you had polio and lost 50 percent of your strength, this is still an easy task to accomplish. After all, you need only 30 percent, so you have 20 percent in reserve. But suppose that through normal aging, disuse, overuse, and perhaps some other factors, you lose 1 to 2 percent of your arm strength per year. If you are gauging your arm strength by how easily you can lift a gallon of milk, you might not even notice this subtle loss of strength for many years. However, when the amount of strength you have lost (from polio and other factors) starts to get close to 20 percent, you will likely notice that lifting a gallon of milk is becoming more difficult. And if one year you are at 30 percent and the next year you drop to 29 percent, you will go from being able to lift the milk to not being able to lift it.

I call this the "all-of-a-sudden" phenomenon because polio survivors tell me that all of a sudden they cannot perform a particular activity. In fact, the loss of strength is not all sudden (it occurs over years), but the inability to do the task frequently does occur all of a sudden. This reserve strength is something we all count on to sustain us as we age. In polio survivors, it is often markedly diminished and contributes to increasing disability that may present without much warning.

So it is easy to see how strength is affected by normal aging, a loss of reserve strength, overuse, and disuse, but what about other medical conditions that affect strength? I generally think of these as being in one of two categories: those that directly cause weakness, such as a compressed nerve in the spine that supplies the leg, or a new problem with the muscles such as a myopathy; and those that do not directly affect the nerves or muscles but cause weakness because they are chronic and generally debilitating. Included in this second category are medications used to treat chronic illnesses that may have side effects that influence strength.

Elaine Fisher is a fifty-nine-year-old woman who had polio at four years of age. Following a six-month hospitalization, she was able to walk with a short left-leg brace. Her right leg, although not as strong as it would have been if she had never had polio, was considered her "good leg." Several months prior to seeing me for the first time, Elaine began complaining of pain, numbness, and tingling in her right leg. At the same time she noticed that it did not feel as sturdy as it had in the past. Elaine had seen her regular doctor several times and had been treated with physical therapy and "increased protein" in her diet. Apparently the presumed diagnosis was PPS. Despite the prescribed treatment, the leg was still painful and not as strong as it had once been.

When I heard Elaine's story, I was immediately suspicious that a problem in her back might be causing pressure on one of the nerves that supplies the muscles in the right leg. I suspected that something other than PPS was to blame for the weakness in the right leg because the numbness and tingling were not symptoms consistent with the diagnosis of PPS. I ordered an MRI (magnetic resonance imaging) study, and it showed a large cyst pressing on her spine and the nerve that supplied the muscles in her leg.

I had several long talks with Elaine about the fact that the cyst was causing her pain and weakness, and that without surgery she might get worse. I sent her to a surgeon, who also recommended surgery as soon as possible. Elaine did not want to risk having the cyst grow and cause further weakness and disability. She underwent surgery on her spine to have it removed and did well postoperatively.

The lesson of this example is that it may be hazardous to assume that new weakness is always due to PPS. New weakness in PPS is a diagnosis of exclusion. Other causes of decreased strength need to be considered first and ruled out, a procedure that is especially critical because many causes of new weakness are treatable and potentially curable.

Chronic medical conditions can sap one's energy and result in generalized fatigue and lack of endurance. The best way to treat this type of weakness is to make sure that the underlying medical condition is optimally treated and that the medications being used are not increasing the fatigue and weakness.

If PPS is determined to be the cause of new weakness, then the treatment is as follows. Rest from activities in which overuse of the muscles may be aggravating the symptoms of weakness. This is often called *relative rest,* meaning that bedrest is not necessary, just avoidance of certain activities. Recognize that simple lifestyle changes may significantly impact your strength. For instance, using a cane for walking may markedly reduce stress on the legs, thereby stopping the downward spiral of leg weakness and perhaps even helping to regain some lost strength. Other examples of relative rest include employing a motorized wheelchair or scooter, using a new brace, and driving with hand controls. The list of possibilities is endless and will be explored in greater depth in later chapters.

Specific exercises may help strengthen the muscles, but they should be done in a supervised and controlled manner under the guidance of polio experts. Some muscles may not be amenable to strengthening, but usually judicious exercise done in a nonfatiguing manner can help improve strength in polio survivors. Appropriate exercises are discussed in Chapter 13.

Medications may help to improve strength; however, there is no "miracle drug." The medication pyridostigmine (Mestinon) promotes chemical reactions at the level of the muscle, which may make muscular contractions stronger in some polio survivors. Any decision to use a medication to help promote strength should be thoroughly discussed with a polio doctor, who can explain the potential risks and benefits as well as monitor the use of the medication.

CHAPTER 9

Fighting Fatigue

Fatigue is the most commonly reported symptom in polio survivors, with more than 90 percent of individuals reporting new or increased fatigue and more than 40 percent disclosing fatigue that interferes with their ability to perform daily activities and work.[1] But polio survivors are not alone in their weariness.

Fatigue is a common complaint to physicians in general practice. In fact, multiple studies have reported that 20 to 40 percent of the general population routinely report feeling fatigued.[2] One can hardly pick up a popular magazine without seeing an article on how to fight fatigue. Yet medical science has learned that fatigue is a key part of the sleep/wake cycles that allow us to rest properly so that when we are awake we can function. If fatigue, then, is a universal and integral part of accomplishing what we need to do each day, when does fatigue become disabling? *When does fatigue cross over from what is normal to what is pathological?*

The usual pattern in humans is to sleep at night and awaken in the morning feeling refreshed and energetic. As the day goes on, our energy level slowly drops and in the evening our fatigue is greatest when we are ready again for sleep. Interspersed in this very general pattern are a lot of other factors that may affect our energy level. For example, if a businesswoman usually eats a light lunch and then goes for a short run during the noon hour, she may feel more energetic than if she goes to a business lunch where she sits for two or three hours and eats a large meal. For the average person, variations in the daily routine do not significantly affect how they are able to function within that routine. When the business lunch is over, the average businesswoman is able to go back to her office and continue work without resting—even if she feels less energetic than in the morning.

We all know from experience that the fatigue produced by extreme physical exertion is different from the fatigue that occurs when we are sedentary. We also know that emotional and psychological factors can affect our energy levels. Stress, anticipation, and excitement may all ultimately make us more tired than usual. Many factors affect our energy levels on any given day.

Fatigue in Post-Polio Syndrome

In studies of polio survivors, fatigue has been the single most commonly reported symptom.[3] Classically, PPS individuals will awaken in the morning feeling refreshed, but will lose that early-morning energy by noon or shortly thereafter. Often there comes a point in the afternoon when they feel overwhelmingly fatigued and are forced to stop and rest. One of the more common descriptions is that a polio survivor feels as though he or she "hits a wall" or "a dark curtain comes down." These descriptions have led researchers to believe that some process is going on that has a physiological basis.

Josephine Maxey is a forty-eight-year-old polio survivor who has had great success as a romance novelist. For years she has been called the "One-a-Day Girl" by her friends and family, because of the fact that she schedules only one major outing each day. For many years

Josephine has experienced disabling fatigue from PPS, which has markedly limited what she is able to accomplish. Josephine has compensated for her reduced energy levels by her scheduling of one activity each day, preferably in the morning when her energy level is highest. She reports with a twinkle in her eye that when her friends call, the first thing they ask is, "Is your One-a-Day booked on such-and-such a date?"

Although Josephine has compensated for years, many persons who complain of fatigue have not adjusted to a different energy level and often are not even sure what "normal" fatigue is. According to a medical dictionary, fatigue is defined as "1) a feeling of tiredness or weariness resulting from continued activity; 2) the state or condition of an organ or tissue in which its response to stimulation is reduced or lost as a result of overactivity."[4]

One way to analyze your own level of fatigue is to answer the following questions:

1. Do you feel tired when you awaken in the morning?
2. Do you have difficulty falling asleep or staying asleep at night?
3. Are you a restless sleeper?
4. Do you snore?
5. Do you feel exhausted during the latter part of the day?
6. Do you stop to rest during the day?
7. Do you take naps during the day?
8. Has your energy level decreased over the past few years?
9. Does fatigue keep you from activities you would like to do?
10. Does fatigue impede your ability to perform your daily routine?
11. Do you have difficulty with memory, concentration, or attention?

If you answered affirmatively to two or more of these questions, then you may have a medical condition that affects your energy level.

The symptom of fatigue in PPS is likely due to the initial virus and its impact on the brain. Called the *central fatigue theory*, this name simply means that the original polio virus affected the central nervous system, including areas in the brain that are responsible for such activities as alertness, concentration, and memory.[5] In support of this theory, researchers have studied the brains of polio survivors and have found evidence suggesting that the polio virus does affect parts of the brain that are associated with wakefulness, attention and memory.[6]

Another theory, which seems plausible but somewhat less likely, is the *peripheral fatigue theory*. It is based on studies which reveal that muscles (which are located in the periphery, as opposed to the brain, which is considered central) are unable continuously to produce a contraction without fatiguing at some point.[7] It makes sense that polio muscles are not as strong as they once were and may be more prone to fatigue after a sustained contraction, but the theory does not explain the problems with memory, concentration, and alertness that many polio survivors report.

Currently, the central theory seems more reasonable because it better coordinates the cognitive symptoms that polio survivors are describing with the anatomical abnormalities that researchers are finding in the brains they have studied. However, the peripheral theory may play a role in PPS fatigue, and neuromuscular fatigue may be part of the fatigue that polio survivors are experiencing. It may be that both the central and peripheral theories are mechanisms which cause fatigue, and that together their effect is more profound than if either one was the sole influence.

Other Medical Causes of Fatigue

Post-Polio Syndrome is not the only medical condition that can cause decreased energy levels. Essentially any chronic medical condition or untreated infection can produce fatigue as a prominent symptom, which in turn can cause further disability and affect one's functioning in the daily routine. Some of the more common medical conditions for which fatigue is a prominent symptom include

Table 9.1 Possible causes of fatigue

Anemia
Anxiety
Cancer and side effects of cancer treatment
Chronic endocrinological illnesses (e.g., diabetes)
Chronic fatigue syndrome
Chronic infection
Chronic pain
Chronic rheumatological illnesses (e.g., rheumatoid arthritis)
Depression
Excessive exercise or muscular overexertion
Fibromyalgia
Heart disease
Hypothyroidism
Illicit drug or alcohol dependency
Overdose or side effects of prescribed medication
Postoperative deconditioning
Post-Polio Syndrome
Postviral infection
Respiratory disorders (e.g., asthma, emphysema)
Sleep disorders (e.g., nocturnal limb movements, obstructive sleep apnea)

thyroid abnormalities, depression, and chronic illnesses such as heart disease and diabetes. Fatigue may also be due to sleep-related medical problems such as sleep apnea (a condition whereby people intermittently stop breathing while they are sleeping). Other respiratory problems can affect energy levels too, as can any type of chronic pain (see Table 9.1).

Because so many medical conditions can influence energy levels, in persons who are experiencing an unusual amount of fatigue it is important to rule out treatable and potentially curable causes of fatigue. For instance, a simple blood test can pick up thyroid problems or anemia (low blood volume), both of which can generate fatigue and can usually be treated with medications. Depression, another common cause of fatigue, can be treated with medications, counseling, or both. It is common for several elements to be contributing at the same time to an individual's fatigue. For instance, someone who is in chronic pain will often use more energy to move about than someone who is not in pain. The extra energy may not be enough to cause noticeable fatigue; however, if the pain affects the quality and quantity of sleep at night, the fatigue may become more prominent. Depression may then become a factor and further exacerbate the fatigue. In order to effectively treat this individual's fatigue, multiple issues need to be considered and a number of interventions may be appropriate.

Joe Klein is an operator of heavy equipment, in his late fifties. He had polio as a child and was left with marked paralysis of his right arm and hand. Joe presented to the polio clinic with symptoms of profound fatigue that was most marked when he got home from work. Although he could function at work, he complained that he had no social life outside work, because his energy levels could not support additional activities. A thorough history, a physical examination, and some simple laboratory blood tests showed Joe's fatigue to be due to multiple factors. These included anemia, sleep apnea, and excessive caffeine and alcohol use.

Anemia can cause fatigue by forcing organs such as the heart to work harder than normal because of reduced blood volume. Sleep apnea can affect the quality of sleep that is a critical part of feeling rejuvenated each day. Caffeine, particularly late in the day, can affect the ability to sleep normally. And alcohol is a known depressant that depletes energy and leaves one feeling sluggish.

Joe was treated with vitamins and iron supplements for his anemia and with a special breathing machine at night for his sleep apnea. He was counseled to avoid caffeine after his midday meal and to try and avoid alcohol altogether. His energy levels improved remarkably with treatment and he began to reclaim his social life. Joe still experiences some fatigue that is probably attributable to PPS; however, it is man-ageable now that the other contributing factors have been rectified.

Treating Fatigue

Effective treatment of fatigue involves the following steps.

> STEP 1. TREATING MEDICAL CONDITIONS THAT MAY
> CAUSE FATIGUE.

The list of medical conditions that can produce fatigue as a symp-tom is extremely long. Therefore, it is important to have a polio doctor recommend what tests should be done in an initial evalua-tion for fatigue in a polio survivor (see Table 9.2 for a list of possible screening tests). Often the polio doctor will work with the primary-care physician, and perhaps other specialists, when attempting to diagnose the basis of the fatigue.

> STEP 2. TREATING SLEEP DISORDERS.

Sleep apnea is found in approximately 40 percent of individuals over the age of sixty-five and is even more common in polio survivors.[8] This topic is of great import and is discussed in detail in Chapter 11. Suffice it to say here that any polio survivor suffering from fatigue, regardless of other symptoms, should have a sleep study to rule out sleep apnea (and other possible sleep disorders).

> STEP 3. TREATING ANXIETY AND DEPRESSION.

Mood disturbances such as anxiety and depression can manifest themselves as fatigue. One clue is when an individual reports that he or she does not feel rested first thing in the morning. With fatigue

Table 9.2 Screening tests that may be done in a fatigue workup

Laboratory blood tests:	complete blood count
	erythrocyte sedimentation rate
	creatinine and urea nitrogen
	glucose
	calcium and phosphorus
	electrolytes
	albumin and total protein
	liver function tests
	thyroid function tests
	rheumatology screen
	C-reactive protein
	viral titers (e.g., Lyme, HIV)
Urinalysis	
Chest x-ray	
Electrocardiogram	
Sleep study	

due to PPS, people usually feel rested in the morning but become progressively fatigued as the day wears on. Therefore, particularly in individuals who report that they fail to feel refreshed in the morning, other causes for fatigue must be investigated. Common causes of early-morning fatigue include mood disturbances and sleep disorders, or in some individuals a combination of both. Certainly not sleeping well can make a person feel frustrated and possibly depressed. On the other hand, someone who is depressed or anxious may not be sleeping well.

In order for symptoms of fatigue to improve, all potential causes must be considered and appropriately treated. Mood disturbances, like PPS, are diagnosed only after other causes of fatigue have been ruled out. In polio survivors who may be adjusting to a new level of disability, it may be difficult to determine how much of their fatigue is caused by discouraged feelings associated with this adjustment and how much is due to a completely separate diagnosis. Because there are so many treatable causes of fatigue (including mood disturbances), a thorough evaluation should be done in persons who are experiencing abnormal levels of fatigue.

STEP 4. CREATING ENERGY-EFFICIENT MOBILITY AND GAIT PATTERNS.

Mobility is an enormous drain on energy. In persons who have altered gait patterns or who are not able to walk at all, mobility may be the single most fatiguing activity that they face. Therefore, energy-efficient mobility and gait patterns are critical in order to limit symptoms of fatigue. This is such an important topic that I have devoted Chapters 18 through 20 to a discussion of how to move from place to place as efficiently as possible.

STEP 5. LIFESTYLE CHANGES IN ORDER TO AVOID MUSCULAR OVERUSE.

Muscular overuse in polio survivors may be a significant source of fatigue. The energy used in mobility is a major drain on polio survivors. Simple daily activities such as driving, ironing, bathing, and the like can also cause fatigue through overuse of the muscles. Chapter 14 explains how to identify and alter activities that are contributing to symptoms of fatigue.

STEP 6. AVOIDING ALCOHOL AND MEDICATIONS THAT CAUSE FATIGUE.

Alcohol is a known depressant that may cause significant fatigue. For anyone who is experiencing fatigue, it is helpful to avoid alcohol as much as possible. Prescription medications, along with nonprescription medications that can be purchased over the counter, may also generate fatigue. It is advisable to review all medications with a knowledgeable physician in order to determine whether they are contributing to symptoms of fatigue. Those that may be causing fatigue perhaps can be discontinued altogether, or replaced by an alternative medication. Obviously, changes in medication regimens should be done only after consulting with a medical doctor.

STEP 7. PRESCRIBING MEDICATIONS FOR POST-POLIO FATIGUE.

The medications that may help to improve symptoms of fatigue fall into two general categories: (1) those used to treat an underlying medical condition that when effectively treated reduces the symptoms of fatigue, and (2) those specifically used to treat post-polio-related fatigue.

In the first category, the list of possible medications is even longer than the list of possible diagnoses (since any given diagnosis may be treated with a variety of medications). For instance, fatigue due to iron-deficiency anemia is best treated with iron supplements. Fatigue due to depression may be treated with antidepressants. Fatigue due to an underactive thyroid gland can be treated with several different thyroid medications. And the list goes on.

In the second category, the list is much shorter. To date no single medication effectively treats symptoms of fatigue in all polio survivors who have PPS. However, there are a few medications that polio survivors and their physicians may want to try. Keep in mind that all medications have potential side effects. Anyone considering medications to help combat post-polio fatigue should discuss the risks and benefits with their polio doctor prior to taking it.

PYRIDOSTIGMINE

Pyridostigmine (also called Mestinon®) is a medication that works at the level of the muscles and was initially thought to be most helpful with muscular overuse fatigue. Unfortunately, clinical trials giving pyridostigmine to polio survivors have had mixed results. Although this substance works well for some polio survivors and should be prescribed accordingly, it is not a miracle drug. Its principal side effects have to do with an increase in bodily secretions, which are generally more uncomfortable than truly dangerous (abdominal cramping and diarrhea may result). Generally these side effects are dose related, and if they appear will resolve with a lower dose. However, polio survivors with significant respiratory problems may not be candidates to try pyridostigmine at all, because it may increase pulmonary secretions.

BROMOCRIPTINE

Bromocriptine (also called Parlodel®) is generally used to treat individuals with Parkinson's disease. This medication works on chemicals in the brain (unlike pyridostigmine, which works on chemicals at the muscle level) and is thought to be potentially helpful with central polio fatigue.[9] Therefore, bromocriptine may help with problems of attention, memory, and concentration. Once again this medication may be very helpful to some individuals with polio, but again is not a miracle drug for everyone. Its most frequently reported side effect is nausea; however, a number of other side effects may be more serious. Anyone considering taking bromocriptine should first consult a doctor.

Other medications that may have provided relief from symptoms of fatigue in some polio survivors include amitryptiline (Elavil®), an antidepressant that may help to establish better sleep patterns; selegiline (Eldepryl®), another medication used to treat Parkinson's disease that acts on chemicals in the brain; and methylphenidate (Ritalin®), which may boost energy levels and improve concentration. (Ritalin is well known for its use in children with problems of attention and concentration.) Further research will undoubtedly bring other medication options to the forefront.

CHAPTER 10

Controlling Cold Intolerance

Although many people complain of sensitivity to or intolerance of cold, polio survivors are more apt to suffer because of injury to nerves that help control the temperature of the body—in particular, the extremities. Atrophied muscles also contribute to the difficulty polio survivors experience when trying to keep their limbs warm, since muscles that do not contract well are unable to assist blood vessels in bringing blood to the extremities. Despite the fact that many polio survivors report that they are sensitive to cold weather and have difficulty keeping their arms and legs warm even under mild weather conditions, most often this is no more than a minor nuisance or inconvenience. Some polio survivors, however, experience very painful and disabling symptoms of cold sensitivity.

Cold intolerance is essentially an uncomfortable feeling, particularly noticeable in the hands and feet, that can cause a coolness which may progress to pain, burning, tingling, stiffness, and changes in skin color.[1] Although anyone may experience cold intolerance in a cold environment, the cold intolerance or sensitivity that occurs in polio survivors is often noticeable indoors in a warm room or is an exaggerated response in a cooler climate.

Polio survivors tend to be more sensitive than other individuals, largely because of injuries to the spinal cord and brain, which are responsible for reacting to climate changes, and because of the peripheral nerves that supply the muscles surrounding the blood vessels that play a large role in warming the extremities.[2] Since the initial polio virus can wreak havoc with the body's ability to adjust to different climates, polio survivors frequently report that they have experienced cold sensitivity since the time of their acute illness. Cold intolerance is also considered to be part of PPS because the symptoms may noticeably worsen years after the initial bout with polio.

Increasing difficulty in regulating the body's temperature (termed *thermoregulation*) is a well-known phenomenon as people age. Scientific studies of injuries and even deaths due to excessive heat or cold environments in the elderly have concluded that many factors play a role.[3] Significantly, older individuals have been shown to have a diminished capacity to adjust to temperature extremes. Sometimes they also have a reduced ability to detect changes in the temperature and therefore may not take steps to help their bodies adjust (such as putting on a sweater or turning up the thermostat). Other studies have focused on the fact that many older individuals live in buildings that are poorly insulated and may not have state-of-the-art heating and air-conditioning systems. Many of them are on fixed incomes and are unwilling or unable to afford to keep their homes at a comfortable temperature. Compounding these problems is the fact that older persons tend to have medical problems (malnutrition, anemia, underactive thyroid function, and so on) that further reduce their ability to regulate their body's temperature.

Polio survivors may experience age-related changes that escalate the preexisting problem of injured nerves and atrophied muscles. Thus, polio survivors who have had some degree of cold sensitivity since their initial illness may experience greater discomfort as they age. In addition to the factors listed above, an accelerated process of nerves "dropping out" may occur (refer to Chapter 2 for further details).

The symptoms of cold intolerance need to be treated, for several reasons. First, it requires an enormous amount of people's energy to try and warm their bodies when they are cold. Second, coordination and mobility are impaired in individuals with cold extremities. And third, the symptoms of cold sensitivity can range from bothersome to excruciatingly painful. Obviously, it is important to provide individuals who are uncomfortable with some relief.

The treatment for cold intolerance or sensitivity is limited to diagnosing and treating any underlying medical conditions such as those described above, and creating a warmer environment for polio survivors who are experiencing symptoms. By that I mean keeping the thermostat turned up, insulating one's home, bundling up with warm clothing, using a commercial heating pad during the day and an electric blanket at night, and other sensible precautions. Keep in mind that particularly when using heating pads or electric blankets there is always the risk of injury if the skin gets too hot. Individuals with peripheral vascular disease should consult their doctor before using any commercial heating devices.

There are no medications, surgeries, or other types of treatment that are recommended exclusively to treat cold intolerance in polio survivors. However, treating medical conditions that contribute to cold sensitivity and creating a warmer environment can provide tremendous relief. Keeping the extremities warm can also improve polio survivors' coordination and mobility, and help them to conserve the body's precious energy.

CHAPTER 11

Respiratory Problems

Respiratory problems in polio survivors could be classified as the great masqueraders, for the symptoms may seem like anything but difficulty in breathing. Before you skip over this chapter because you breathe well and assume you have no respiratory problems, bear in mind that respiratory conditions may be subtle, may not have to do with breathing when you are awake, and may have nothing to do with whether you had respiratory problems during the initial polio episode. I admit to having neglected respiratory issues in polio survivors in the past. Over the years, however, I have gained new respect for how often respiratory conditions are at the root of polio survivors' complaints (of fatigue, depressed mood, headaches, and the like). Moreover, I am impressed by how amenable many of these conditions are to treatment—particularly in individuals who do not have marked difficulty breathing during the day.

One of the primary reasons that polio survivors may be at risk for problems with respiratory function is that with normal aging everyone's respiratory status declines somewhat.[1] In individuals who have normal lungs and respiratory muscles, the age-related changes in respiratory function are hardly noticeable. Unfortunately, the same may not be true for polio survivors, who often have significantly less reserve strength in their respiratory muscles owing to the initial polio. Regardless of whether a polio survivor had significant breathing problems during the original infection, a subtle loss of respiratory muscle strength can result in new respiratory problems that require medical intervention.[2]

Although it is difficult to control the normal age-related decline in respiratory function, certain factors can be modified. For example, smoking can exacerbate any underlying breathing problems and cause significant new problems such as chronic obstructive pulmonary disease (COPD) and lung cancer. Quitting smoking can certainly improve respiratory status. Moreover, individuals who are overweight may improve their breathing problems by losing weight. Scoliosis and certain postural conditions may also aggravate breathing problems; therefore, improving one's posture when seated or standing can help with respiratory difficulties.

Another reason why polio survivors are at risk for new respiratory problems is that the initial polio may have injured the brain's respiratory control center. Studies have shown that polio survivors are at risk for sleep apnea—a problem that may arise from how the brain regulates breathing.[3]

Symptoms Associated with Underlying Respiratory Problems

Too often both polio survivors and the medical professionals who treat them fail to recognize the early signs of respiratory problems. Early symptoms may be subtle and not easily associated with respiratory function. The symptoms may come on so gradually that they seem hardly noticeable until the afflicted person takes time to reflect on how he or she felt a decade or more ago. Polio survivors and physicians who treat polio survivors need to be diligent about exploring the possibility of respiratory decline in individuals presenting with a variety of new symptoms.

Frequently, the earliest signs of problems with respiratory function include headaches (particularly awakening with a headache), fatigue, nightmares, restless or interrupted sleep, difficulty sleeping while lying down, poor concentration, anxiety, and inability to speak loudly or without stopping frequently to take a breath. People with more conspicuous respiratory problems may notice shortness of breath with exertion, frequent respiratory infections, and a general feeling of not breathing adequately. Individuals who have required continuous breathing support since their initial polio may notice a change in ventilator settings, an inability to effectively use equipment that has worked well for them in the past, and a general worsening of their overall respiratory status. Regardless of whether the symptoms are obvious or subtle, it is crucial to evaluate respiratory function in all polio survivors who are experiencing new problems.

Respiratory Evaluation

Evaluation by a physician who is an expert in polio and PPS is the first step in determining what might be causing any new or worsening problems in polio survivors. Polio doctors in general have a high level of suspicion that a decline in respiratory function may cause the symptoms listed above, and they can selectively order appropriate tests or suggest a pulmonary specialist for further evaluation. Although some polio survivors may want every test imaginable to work up their symptoms and others may want to undergo as few tests as possible, the most reasonable approach is for a pulmonologist with expertise in polio-related respiratory disorders to recommend the tests that are most likely to facilitate the correct diagnosis.

CHRONIC ALVEOLAR HYPOVENTILATION

Two respiratory conditions are commonly seen in polio survivors. The first is a weakness of the respiratory muscles that does not allow proper gas exchange (of oxygen and carbon dioxide) in the lungs. This is called *chronic alveolar hypoventilation* (CAH). The typical workup for CAH includes a series of laboratory tests (including blood tests and breathing tests).[4]

As noted above, CAH is a disorder that involves poor exchange of the oxygen that the body needs with the carbon dioxide that the body wants to get rid of. The cause of CAH in polio survivors is weakened muscles. Therefore, the treatment involves assisting the respiratory muscles to facilitate this gas exchange, most often by using a ventilatory device during sleep. (This procedure can dramatically improve how one feels during the day.) The device most commonly used is called a Bi-PAP, which stands for bilevel positive airway pressure. A CPAP (continuous positive airway pressure) device is sometimes used, but may not be as effective in treating CAH. Note that supplemental oxygen is generally not useful and may indeed be harmful.

The several ways to use Bi-PAP all involve wearing some sort of mask over the nose or face (Figure 11.1). In most instances Bi-PAP will treat CAH effectively as long as the individual can tolerate wearing a mask (generally during sleep) and the mask fits well.[5]

Other treatments include the use of various ventilators, a rocking bed, a pneumobelt, and a tracheostomy.[6] All are considered noninvasive treatments—with the exception of a tracheostomy, in which a small tube is surgically inserted into the trachea. A detailed description of these treatments is beyond the scope of this chapter.

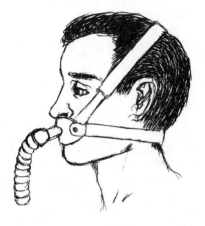

Fig. 11.1. Intermittent positive pressure ventilation through the mouth.

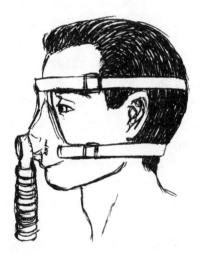

Fig. 11.2. Intermittent positive pressure ventilation through the nose.

SLEEP APNEA

The second common respiratory problem in polio survivors is *sleep apnea,* defined as "an intermittent cessation of airflow at the nose and mouth during sleep."[7] During sleep, the breathing stops altogether for a period, over and over again. The time when the individual is not breathing may be as short as ten seconds or as long as two to three minutes. Frequently, people with sleep apnea will have ten to fifteen periods (or more) each hour when they stop breathing. Sleep apnea is one of the most common causes of daytime fatigue and is nearly always treatable. It can be classified as obstructive, central, or a mix of the two. All of these types may be found in polio survivors.[8]

In obstructive sleep apnea, because of a mechanical problem in the airway the air simply cannot get through. Generally the difficulty occurs at the level of the upper airway. Someone with obstructive sleep apnea may stop breathing four hundred to five hundred times each night! Alcohol and obesity both make the symptoms of obstructive sleep apnea significantly worse. Scientific studies have implicated obstructive sleep apnea in high blood pressure, heart attack, stroke, and even sudden death.[9]

Central sleep apnea is caused by a malfunction in the brain that temporarily turns off the signals that control breathing. It often occurs together with CAH. Obesity is not as common a factor in central sleep apnea as it is in obstructive sleep apnea.

Polio survivors should be suspicious of sleep apnea if they have any of the following symptoms: daytime fatigue, snoring at night, or episodes where someone else has witnessed that they stopped breathing or choked or gasped during sleep. Other factors that may predict (but not necessarily cause) sleep apnea include a history of high blood pressure or CAH, restless sleep, mood changes, difficulty with memory and concentration (intellectual function), being over-weight (even moderately), and morning headaches.

The diagnosis of sleep apnea is generally made after a sleep study is performed (polysomnography). Treatment depends on the results and takes into account the individual's symptoms and physical examination. In general, treatment may include avoiding sleeping on one's back, oral medications, weight reduction, avoiding alcohol, wearing appliances at night (such as a mouth guard), surgery to improve mechanical problems (correcting a deviated nasal septum), and nighttime use of ventilatory appliances such as a CPAP. Supplemental oxygen may or may not be useful.

OTHER CAUSES

Although CAH and sleep apnea are the most common respiratory conditions found in polio survivors, other factors may affect respiratory function. For instance, a lung condition called chronic obstructive pulmonary disease is common in smokers and may cause a person to feel short of breath. Or the individual's heart may not be functioning properly. Someone else may have an underlying pneumonia that needs to be treated. Still another reason may be atelectasis (a condition in which the lungs do not fully inflate) after a period of being bedridden (perhaps during recovery from a minor surgical procedure or an illness). The list of possibilities is long. Therefore, any polio survivor experiencing a change in breathing or respiratory status (or who has any of the other symptoms described in this chapter) should be evaluated.

Respiratory problems are much more common in polio survivors than is often recognized. The symptoms may be subtle, or they may not be thought to be associated with a respiratory disorder (such as fatigue or morning headaches). I routinely recommend baseline pulmonary function tests, and often other tests such as sleep studies. I am impressed by the dramatic change in symptoms when underlying respiratory problems (including CAH and sleep apnea) are appropriately treated. Often people experience significant improvement in fatigue, intellectual function, daytime breathing, mood, and even pain. Clearly, a vigilant approach to diagnosing and treating respiratory disorders in polio survivors can significantly better their quality of life.

CHAPTER 12

Swallowing Issues

My grandfather was a polio survivor who had profound difficulty with swallowing that progressed as he aged. Although not all polio survivors who develop swallowing problems have had bulbar polio (which affects the muscles that control swallowing and breathing), my grandfather did have this type. He was typical of many bulbar polio survivors in that his recovery from the initial polio left little evidence that he had ever had any problems with breathing or swallowing. Yet his later years were punctuated with coughing, throat clearing, and downright choking during every meal.

I distinctly recall that one of my grandfather's greatest pleasures was to take his children and grandchildren out to eat. Although he favored small restaurants (some my mother called *greasy diners*), they were comfortable and familiar establishments where he knew the menus and enjoyed the food and companionship of family. My first memories of these outings with Pa Pa are that, as a very young child, I and my siblings were assigned the job of looking for a "paralyzed parking" space for his van (this term I assume my grandfather taught us because his legs were paralyzed from the original polio). I have memories of waitresses at some later time asking my elder brother or me what my grandfather wanted to eat. Apparently they assumed that because he used a wheelchair, he was unable to order for himself. We would look over at my grandfather in confusion, and he would politely order his meal.

My adult memories of dining with my grandfather are overshadowed by his valiant and often painful struggle to swallow his food. I was in college when I first noticed that Pa Pa frequently coughed and cleared his throat while eating. By the time I was in medical school he was gagging on his food, and this progressed to choking when he ate. Startled restaurant patrons would perch on the edge of their seats, certain they would soon be needed to provide resuscitation or at the very least to call 911. As calmly and unobtrusively as we could manage, my brother and sister and I would eat our own meals and chat with each other. Eating was such a struggle for my grandfather that he was unable to participate in the conversation. Still, he took me out to eat every time I came home to visit.

At some point I urged my mother to have my grandfather evaluated for his swallowing. (My grandfather was not fond of going to doctors, so this was a touchy subject that always was delegated to my mother, who could usually charm my grandfather into going.) Not surprisingly, the tests revealed that the muscles involved in swallowing were not working well. Nor were they working in a coordinated manner. Moreover, food and liquids were routinely going down the wrong tube. When food goes down the trachea instead of the esophagus, this is called *aspiration*. Aspirating food and drink can be very dangerous and may lead to death by choking or by causing pneumonia in the lungs. The concerned doctor convinced my grandfather to have a feeding tube placed in his stomach through which he could receive all of his nutrition. Stubborn and proud, my grandfather refused to use his feeding tube. Until he eventually died of unrelated causes, he continued to eat—aspirating the entire time.

My grandfather had the worst swallowing problems I have ever seen in a polio survivor. He essentially refused medical treatment, in part because he was not inclined to complain but also because he did not have faith in the health-care professionals involved in his care, none of whom had any significant experience with polio survivors. I was just beginning my medical career at the time, and my ability to help him was limited.

Swallowing and Polio

The majority of polio survivors do not have the kind of profound swallowing problems that my grandfather experienced. In most instances, they are more like my mother (also a polio survivor, who reportedly did not have bulbar polio) who clears her throat more often than others, loses her voice with nearly every cold she gets, and sleeps poorly. What does all of this mean with respect to polio survivors and swallowing? Coughing, choking, and throat clearing are all signs that someone may be having difficulty with swallowing (termed *dysphagia*). Difficulty raising one's voice, a raspy voice, or regular loss of one's voice are all signs that there may have been injury to the vocal cords (laryngeal muscles) during the initial polio.[1] Sleeping fitfully, snoring, and early-morning fatigue are all signs that sleep apnea or other sleep disorders may be present in polio survivors (review Chapters 9 and 11 for details). I mention all of these symptoms together because swallowing, speech, and breathing problems often occur simultaneously in polio survivors. The nerves and muscles that control these functions are in close proximity and may all have been affected to varying degrees during the initial polio—even if bulbar polio was not thought to be present.

In fact, one study reported that nearly one in five polio survivors will experience problems with swallowing which may run the gamut from hardly noticeable to severe and potentially life threatening.[2] The number of polio survivors experiencing swallowing problems may actually be much higher; the one-in-five figure may reflect the fact that polio survivors are not reporting swallowing problems, either because they fail to notice them or because they have learned to adjust to these problems as minor issues. Polio survivors who initially had swallowing and respiratory complications are more likely to have difficulty with swallowing; however, even those survivors who did not have bulbar polio initially may be at risk for dysphagia as they age.[3] Swallowing problems in polio survivors tend to progress fairly slowly, and persons who are treated appropriately can almost always avoid serious complications.[4]

The risks associated with untreated swallowing problems are well known. We have seen that food and liquids can go down the wrong tube (the trachea) and cause choking or aspiration of these substances into the lungs. Aspirated food can lodge in the airways when one tries to swallow, a blockage that can lead to sudden loss of the ability to breathe. Difficulty in swallowing may also be associated with problems controlling oral secretions (saliva) and may result in drooling.

SWALLOWING PROBLEMS THAT ARE DISABLING

Persons with swallowing problems may feel intensely anxious about eating. They may isolate themselves and eat only when no one else is present, because of their embarrassment. Other persons with dysphagia may insist on eating only when others are present, feeling that their difficulty swallowing is potentially life threatening and they may need resuscitation if they choke. In the first instance, the quality of life is negatively impacted because of social withdrawal and isolation. In the second scenario, the quality of life is affected because of loss of independence and inability to choose when and where to eat regardless of who else is present. Thus, even though the symptoms of dysphagia may not be severe, their impact may lead to feelings of anxiety and depression.

Dysphagia may be formally classified as a handicap when it interferes with a person's ability to enjoy eating and sharing meals with other people.[5] In some instances, it may affect the entire life situation including ability to exercise, work in a specific environment, and participate in meaningful leisure activities. While it may seem drastic to classify dysphagia as a handicap, we know that eating does much more than satiate our appetites. Food has symbolic meaning and provides comfort and feelings of community involvement; it may even be part of our religious and ethnic life. Consequently, untreated swallowing problems may significantly affect people's lives—even if they are not at serious risk of choking or aspirating.

SWALLOWING AND OTHER MEDICAL CONDITIONS

As noted earlier, swallowing problems in polio survivors may be associated with other medical problems as well. The most serious of these are the respiratory problems, which have been discussed in detail in the previous chapter. The muscles involved in speaking may also have been affected by the initial polio and may become weaker as one ages. The result can be problems with voice quality, pitch, and loudness. Individuals whose laryngeal muscles have been affected often complain that their voices "tire" and that they are reduced to whispering and straining when talking. Moreover, they may be susceptible to repeated episodes of laryngitis.

Another potential issue associated with swallowing problems is weight loss or weight gain. It makes sense that if people cannot swallow well, they probably have a tendency to eat less and therefore lose weight. Counterintuitively, the opposite may be true: sometimes persons with dysphagia actually gain weight because in order to feel satiated they tend to eat small, frequent meals that are high in calories. Although these can keep one's energy at an appropriate level, they will only do so if they contain carefully selected low-fat foods that are nutritious (see Chapter 15).

Swallowing problems may masquerade as heart disease when they present with heartburn or chest pain. Although heart disease is often associated with shortness of breath and sweating, these symptoms may not be present. When chest pain is the sole symptom, the etiology of the pain may be heart disease or swallowing problems. Another possibility is gastroesophageal reflux disease (GERD), which occurs when the acidic contents of the stomach back up into the esophagus and cause irritation that leads to "heartburn." The possibility of genuine heart disease is the most alarming and should be considered the first priority of assessment. If no serious problems with the cardiovascular system are uncovered and the symptoms of chest pain and/or heartburn continue, the next organ system to evaluate is the gastrointestinal. Examination should include evaluation for dysphagia and gastroesophageal reflux. In some individuals more than one problem may be present. Therefore, even if there is evidence of heart disease in polio survivors that may account for symptoms of chest pain and heartburn, the possibility of concomitant swallowing problems should also be entertained.

SWALLOWING AND NORMAL AGING

Polio survivors are not alone in being at risk for swallowing problems. Research reveals that in the general aging population, the risk of developing swallowing problems is considerable.[6] In one study, 35 percent of men and women (ages fifty to seventy-nine) complained of swallowing and esophageal problems.[7] Because dysphagia is often associated with medical conditions that are treatable and potentially curable, neither aging nor Post-Polio Syndrome should be considered the cause of dysphagia until other diagnoses have

Table 12.1 Medical illnesses that may have associated swallowing problems

---

Bulbar poliomyelitis and Post-Polio Syndrome
Stroke
Traumatic brain injury
Myasthenia gravis
Infection or abscess
Multiple sclerosis
Amyotrophic lateral sclerosis
Autoimmune disease (e.g., scleroderma, dermatomyositis, Sjogren's)
Diabetes mellitus
Spinal arthritis
Muscular dystrophy
Myopathy
Diverticula
Structural constriction due to strictures, rings, and webs in the esophagus
Postoperative complications of head and neck surgery
Gastroesophageal reflux disease (GERD)
Vocal-cord paralysis
Lyme disease
Head and neck cancer
Peritonsillar abscess
Tetanus
Bell's palsy
Postnasal drip
Drug or alcohol abuse

Note: The list above gives examples of medical conditions that may have swallowing problems associated with them. It is not a complete list.

been reviewed and ruled out. Some of the more common medical conditions associated with dysphagia are listed in Table 12.1.

The prevalence of swallowing problems and their association with a variety of medical conditions (as well as with "normal" aging) has prompted intense interest in the medical and scientific communities. Research endeavors increasingly have focused on the evaluation and treatment of dysphagia. The result has been more sophisticated diagnostic and treatment options, and it is likely that this trend will continue.

Normal and Abnormal Swallowing

Typically, people swallow about six hundred times a day.[8] More than forty paired muscles work in concert to make this an effortless endeavor. The normal swallow has multiple phases that start in the mouth and propel saliva, food, and liquids to the stomach by way of the esophagus. The early stages of swallowing are voluntary and may be affected by taste, food preferences, food textures, and satiation. Once the food gets to the esophageal level, however, the remainder of the swallow is essentially an involuntary reflex. In a normal swallow, both food and liquids are managed easily without coughing or choking.

Problems may occur anywhere along the path from the mouth through the esophagus to the stomach. The term *dysphagia* is rather nonspecific and simply means that a problem is occurring at some level in the process. At the start of the swallow, what is termed the oral preparatory phase, it may be that food or liquid leaks out of the mouth. As the swallow progresses, there may be symptoms of coughing, choking, or feeling as though there is a lump in the throat. In more severe cases, the contents of the mouth may be propelled down the trachea instead of the esophagus.

The severity of symptoms in dysphagia often reflects the severity of the problem, but not always. People with mild symptoms may not even recognize that they have a swallowing problem, and people with very severe symptoms may continually aspirate (termed *silent aspiration*) without realizing it. The symptoms of dysphagia may include coughing, choking, and regurgitation. Table 12.2 gives a more comprehensive list of the commonly encountered symptoms.

Table 12.2 Symptoms of dysphagia

Drooling
Difficulty removing food from an eating utensil
Difficulty chewing
Biting the tongue
Excessive tongue motions
Multiple swallows required to move food down
Food or liquid coming out of the nose (nasal regurgitation)
Food or pills sticking in the throat
Choking
Excessive clearing of the throat
Feeling a lump in the throat
Coughing
Breathy or nasal voice
Hoarseness after swallowing
Gurgling wet voice
Difficulty taking part in conversations at mealtime
Difficulty reaching satiety
Feeling hungry or thirsty after a meal
Heartburn
Avoidance of certain foods or liquids
Feelings of anxiety when eating
Excessive time required to complete a meal (e.g., more than 40 minutes)
Unexplained weight loss or weight gain

Note: These symptoms are not diagnostic of dysphagia and may be found in other medical conditions.

Even without obvious evidence of swallowing problems, other clues may hint that dysphagia is present. For instance, dysphagia might be suspected in someone who feels anxious about swallowing. Specifically in polio survivors, dysphagia should be suspected in anyone who is experiencing respiratory problems or having difficulty with voice tone, pitch, and articulation (because of the close proximity of the breathing, speech, and swallowing muscles). Recognizing the symptoms is the essential first step in diagnosing and treating dysphagia.

Evaluation of Abnormal Swallowing

The goals of a swallowing evaluation are as follows: (1) establish the correct diagnosis, (2) evaluate the location and severity of the problem, (3) address the individual's nutritional status, and (4) recommend appropriate treatment. A qualified specialist who treats dysphagia will go through a three-step process. The first is to take an oral history, specifically to identify what symptoms the individual is experiencing. Some of the questions the specialist may ask are, Do you have any symptoms of coughing when you eat or drink? Do you have episodes of choking? Do you have any heartburn? Do you feel anxious when you eat? Are you more likely to experience symptoms when you are tired? Also during this part of the evaluation, the specialist will obtain a complete list of the individual's current medications, and information regarding past medical problems that may have affected the head and neck (tracheotomy, stroke, and the like).

The second step in the evaluation is the physical examination. This may include general observation of an individual's posture, alertness, and voice quality and pitch. The specialist will also palpate the structures of the individual's upper body, focusing on the head and neck. Medical instruments may be employed to visualize areas that are difficult to examine: perhaps specially designed mirrors, similar to what a dentist uses to examine the mouth and throat; or a more sophisticated instrument called an endoscope, to examine deeper structures in the throat (such as the esophagus or vocal cords).

The third step of the evaluation involves special tests and studies to rule out or confirm specific diagnoses. These may be laboratory (blood) tests and different types of x-ray studies. Table 12.3 lists some of the more common tests used to visualize the swallowing process. One frequently utilized test is the modified barium swallow. Barium is placed in food or liquids and used as a tracer. The patient swallows

Table 12.3 Diagnostic imaging studies used to evaluate dysphagia

Modified barium swallow
Functional endoscopic evaluation of swallowing
Videofluorography
Fiberoptic nasoendoscopy
Manography
Ultrasonography
Endoscopy

Note: It is beyond the scope of this chapter to describe the various swallowing tests and how they are performed. If a particular test is recommended for an individual, the details should be discussed ahead of time with the prescribing specialist.

Table 12.4 Examples of treatments for dysphagia

Swallowing maneuvers and techniques (e.g., supraglottic swallow, dry swallow after each bite, effortful swallow)
Head and neck maneuvers (e.g., chin tuck, head rotation, head tilt)
Posture adjustments (e.g., improving sitting posture, addressing scoliosis)
Appropriate meal times and variation of food consistencies (e.g., alternating liquids and solids, drinking thickened liquids)
Oral motor exercises
Medication additions or deletions
Injections (e.g., botulinum toxin)
Biofeedback
Thermal stimulation
Antireflux treatment (e.g., treat GERD)
Surgery
Assessment of nutritional status
Alternative feeding routes (generally only in very severe cases, through a tube placed in the stomach or small intestine)

Note: Not all of these treatments are applicable to PPS. Appropriate treatment should be undertaken only after consultation with skilled specialists.

the barium-laced food or drink and the entire swallowing process is visualized by means of a special x-ray technique. This test allows a specialist to see exactly where problems are occurring and whether any of the barium is going down the trachea and into the lungs. It is an easy test to administer and can provide a great deal of valuable information; thus, it is often one of the first tests ordered. Another commonly ordered test is the functional endoscopic evaluation of swallowing, which involves placing a special scope at the back of the nose and then watching the individual ingest food and liquids.

Deciding which tests to utilize to evaluate a given individual's swallowing problems is best left to the discretion of a specialist. More than one consultant may be asked to participate in the diagnostic workup and treatment. For example, a medical doctor who specializes in dysphagia may collaborate with a speech and language pathologist, who can provide valuable input.

Once the evaluation is completed and an appropriate diagnosis is made, the final step is to recommend treatment options. These will vary markedly depending on precisely what is causing the difficulties and where in the swallowing process the problems are occurring. Treatment options will also reflect the specialist's prior experience and successful strategies and the polio survivor's willingness to pursue a variety of options. Table 12.4 gives the reader an idea of the treatment possibilities. In no way does this chapter substitute for evaluation by a medical specialist, and under no circumstances should treatment be considered without the advice and counsel of a specialist. Moreover, the scope of treatment should be based on the individual's specific complaints, diagnosis, and interest in pursuing treatment.

CHAPTER 13

Exercise Essentials

Many individuals who contracted polio during the epidemics have spent a lifetime guided by the words "Use it or lose it"—a philosophy instilled in them during their initial illness by physical therapists and physicians who believed exercise to be critical in recovering from acute paralytic polio. However, people who had polio decades ago are now hearing the exact opposite: "Use it and you *will* lose it." Even published studies have not provided consistent guidelines. The topic of exercise has become one of the most confusing issues for polio survivors as they age. Research during the 1990s indicated that exercise in polio survivors is beneficial if done appropriately. Experts agree that, in general, polio survivors should exercise—in a controlled and judicious manner.[1] The discussion in this chapter applies to all persons with a history of polio, irrespective of whether they have been diagnosed with Post-Polio Syndrome.

The Exercise Controversy

The controversy is actually fairly simple to understand, but far more complicated to address. The main concern is that *overuse of the muscles may lead to further weakness, which may be permanent.* It is a frightening thought for those who are already having difficulty doing the activities they formerly were able to accomplish easily. At this point polio survivors may be thinking, "Why risk exercising?" The answer is, Because the benefits greatly outweigh the risks. And the risks can be minimized if one exercises properly.

Despite the controversy, most experts agree that an appropriate exercise regimen should be tailored to individual polio survivors based on their needs and a physical examination. In muscles that are quite weak (a reasonable test is to see whether the muscle can be contracted against the force of gravity), the general guideline is to perform nonfatiguing exercise. Stronger muscles can handle more aggressive exercise. A simple concept on the surface, in practice it becomes quite challenging to stay within the boundaries of non-fatiguing exercise. Fatigue is a subjective experience, dependent on interpretation by the individual. It is difficult to measure, so individuals are responsible for reporting when they feel tired. Just as some people have high (or low) levels of pain tolerance, so do some polio survivors have high (or low) fatigue levels.

Another potential stumbling block in designing appropriate exercise programs for polio survivors is that some individuals have been taught to persevere despite feelings of fatigue and even pain. Polio expert Lauro Halstead has written of his own experience with polio, and the denial mechanisms that have both helped and hindered him throughout his life. Dr. Halstead compares polio survivors to marathon runners. Both push themselves to their limits, often ignoring fatigue, pain, and suffering. Using Halstead's analogy, the historian Hugh Gallagher wrote in the magazine *New Mobility*: "Runners are odd people. They are focused, even obsessed, with their running. They run every day and neither snow nor rain nor dark of night will stop them. They drive themselves to extraordinary feats of endurance, forcing their bodies to perform far beyond normal capacities. And as they age, it gets tougher and tougher for them to keep at it. They never give up. They are stubborn people who refuse to accept their limitations. And so are we. Our muscles are fully or partially paralyzed. They have only a fraction of normal strength and endurance. Nevertheless, we have taught them to perform marvelous feats. With exercise, ingenuity and a good deal of chicanery, we have found ways to make our muscles perform what are for others the simplest tasks of daily living."[2]

If polio survivors are constantly pushing themselves to their limits to perform daily activities, the obvious question is whether additional formal exercise routines will be detrimental. In some instances, perhaps; in many other instances, however, a supervised exercise program can be quite helpful. Increasing strength and endurance through exercise has the potential to make daily activities seem more like a 10K than a marathon. Nonetheless, the issues surrounding exercise are so complex that an exercise program should never be undertaken without the judicious guidance of experts.

The Goals of Exercise

Any exercise program may include some or all of the following as its goals: (1) improve *strength*; (2) improve *flexibility*; (3) improve *endurance*; and (4) improve *coordination*.

Each goal requires specific exercises, and an ideal regimen will incorporate exercises that address all of the goals. Still, not all of the goals are equally important to a given individual, and the amount of time spent on each activity should reflect what one hopes to accomplish. The following examples are designed to highlight differences in exercise protocols based on the individual's specific needs. Keep in mind as you read them that most exercise programs ideally incorporate all four basic components, and that these examples are meant to demonstrate the adaptation of a program to meet specific needs.

EXERCISING TO IMPROVE STRENGTH

A minimum amount of strength is necessary to do any given task. Many polio survivors exert a great deal of strength to perform the tasks of their daily routine. Because they are functioning at near-maximal levels, even a small change in strength can cause a noticeable change in function. For example, one polio survivor told me that at the start of a cold New England winter he was no longer able to put on his winter coat. The previous winter he had struggled, but had been able to put the same coat on. The next year, it was simply too heavy and cumbersome. Although there was no significant change in strength testing on his physical examination, he was noticing signs of increased weakness during his daily activities. Despite a rather subtle change in strength, he had encountered a rather marked change in his ability to dress himself for the cold weather.

Polio survivors often are understandably discouraged when a small change in strength prevents them from doing something they previously had been able to do. Fortunately, the opposite is also true: a small gain in strength can mean a great improvement in the ability to function.

Strengthening exercises have been one of the most controversial topics in exercise for polio survivors. There is legitimate concern that such exercises may unnecessarily strain muscles that are already working very hard. Despite the potential for further weakness, studies show that strengthening exercises can safely be done by most polio survivors if performed judiciously under the guidance of experts.[3]

Mary Constantine is a sixty-year-old polio survivor who recently had surgery to release a pinched nerve at her wrist (carpal tunnel syndrome). Mary has relied heavily on her strong arms to compensate for the weakness in her legs. Even after her surgery she continued to have difficulty grasping objects and opening jars. Her orthopedic surgeon assured her that her surgery had been a success. When Mary came to the polio clinic, it was evident that she needed to do some gentle strengthening exercises to improve the weakness that was caused by both the pinched nerve and the fact that she had been favoring her injured hand for months (often called disuse weakness*). After working with an occupational therapist skilled in treating polio survivors, Mary found her hand strength improving substantially.*

Strengthening exercises are based on the *overload principle,* which essentially means that in order to improve the strength in any given muscle, it must be sufficiently challenged or overloaded. In other words, muscles increase in strength and size when they are forced to contract at maximal or near-maximal levels. This seems inherently to violate the concept of a *nonfatiguing* exercise program. How can one overload one's muscles in order to build strength, yet not fatigue those same muscles? Despite numerous medical studies, the answer is still ambiguous. Therefore, strengthening exercises in polio survivors must be performed with particular caution and should be carefully prescribed by a physician (refer to Table 13.1 for the outline of a typical exercise prescription form).

Strengthening exercises involve two important features: *resistance* and *repetitions.* Resistance is the amount of weight or tension required to perform the exercise, and repetitions are the number of times the exercise is done. Both elements must be carefully monitored in a strengthening program for polio survivors.

Although the strength of the muscles is a primary consideration in defining the limits of a strengthening program, electromyography and nerve conduction studies (commonly called EMG and described in Chapter 5) may be helpful.[4] These studies can help answer the following questions: Is there evidence of old polio in all extremities or have some been spared? Is there evidence that the muscles and nerves are suffering a new injury, either from overuse or

Table 13.1 Sample exercise prescription form

Name
Diagnosis
Precautions (e.g., nonfatiguing program)
Type of exercise (e.g., isometric)
Duration of exercise (e.g., length of time, repetitions, sets)
Frequency of exercise (e.g., how many times each week)
Intensity of exercise (e.g., resistance, tension)

Note: The typical structure of an exercise session is as follows: warm-up, stretching, main task (e.g., swimming, weight training), and cool-down.

from a distinctly separate nerve or muscle injury? If the extremities are clinically very strong (test normal on manual muscle testing during physical examination) and do not show any evidence of old polio, exercise recommendations can be much more liberal and allow a more aggressive strengthening program.

EXERCISING TO IMPROVE FLEXIBILITY

Flexibility exercises are designed to increase the range of motion in the extremities, neck, and trunk. Muscles, tendons, and ligaments have a tendency to contract or get shorter when they are not stretched regularly, thereby restricting the range of motion at a particular joint such as the ankle or in the neck or trunk. Poor range of motion can be painful, disabling, and sometimes dangerous. For example, someone with neck pain may not want to turn their head to the side because the motion hurts too much. After a short period (days to weeks) it becomes difficult to turn the head because the muscles, tendons, and ligaments have not been stretched regularly. Often the result is even more pain and an impact on the ability to perform routine tasks (such as driving, where turning one's head when switching lanes is critical for safety).

In polio survivors, tight heel cords notoriously cause problems; they increase the amount of energy required to walk, and potentially cause falls as it becomes more difficult for the foot to clear when walking. Lack of flexibility is also a major culprit in back pain, which may be completely eliminated by improving flexibility in the trunk and legs.

Jane Black is a fifty-year-old polio survivor who, despite having some residual paralysis in her left leg, has never had to use braces or assistive devices to ambulate. When Jane first came to the polio clinic, she was concerned that she could no longer function professionally. She works as an interior designer and was having increased difficulty at clients' homes, where she would trip on uneven surfaces and carpet thresholds. Her initial evaluation yielded some obvious clues to the reason. She had lost some of the range of motion in her ankles, and particularly on the left side was not able to clear her foot well when trying to swing it through. The left foot would get caught, and Jane would stumble. After a short course of physical therapy, her ankles were much more flexible and she was no longer tripping. Not only was Jane walking better, she was using less energy when she ambulated.

Flexibility exercises are a critical but often neglected part of any exercise program. Some people are remarkably flexible without much effort, while others are quite inflexible. Even these people can improve their flexibility with appropriate exercise. Figures 13.1 to 13.10, with Table 13.2, give examples of simple stretches that nearly all polio survivors can safely perform.

In general, flexibility exercises involve both *active* and *passive* stretching. The difference may seem obvious, but is actually quite important. Active stretching is done by the individual, whereas passive stretching involves someone else performing the stretches on the individual. These terms have led to confusion in the polio literature.

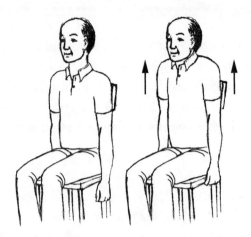

Fig. 13.1. Shoulder shrug: This exercise helps to relax and strengthen neck muscles as well as improve posture. 1. Sit or lie down with your arms relaxed at your side. 2. Shrug your shoulders as high as possible toward your ears. Take a deep breath while raising your shoulders and exhale as you relax. 3. Repeat 5 times.

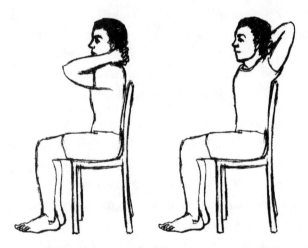

Fig. 13.2. Chicken wing: This exercise helps to improve posture and range of motion in the shoulders and chest muscles. 1. You can do this exercise sitting or standing. 2. Place your hands behind your head with elbows in front. 3. Move your elbows back as far as possible. Keep your chin in and your head back. You should feel a gentle stretch in your chest. Hold this position for 5 seconds. 4. Return to the starting position and repeat 5 times.

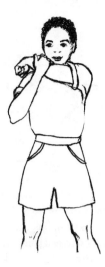

Fig. 13.3. Posterior capsule shoulder stretch: This exercise helps stretch out the shoulder.

1. You can do this exercise sitting, standing, or lying down.
2. Gently pull your elbow with the opposite hand until you feel a stretch in your shoulder.
3. Hold this position for 5 seconds.
4. Repeat 5 times and then do this stretch on the other arm.

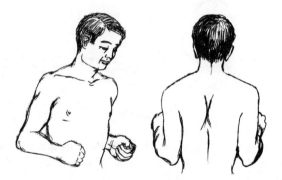

Fig. 13.4. Shoulder blade squeeze: This exercise helps to stretch your chest and shoulder muscles, strengthen your shoulder muscles, and improve posture.

1. Sit or stand as tall as possible.
2. Pull your shoulders back, squeezing your shoulder blades together. Try to get your elbows as close together as possible behind your back.
3. Hold this position for 5 seconds and repeat 5 times.

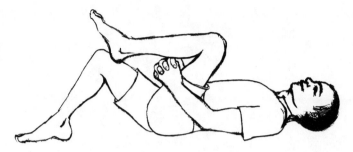

Fig. 13.5. Single knee to chest stretch: This exercise helps to stretch out your hamstring muscles in the back of your leg as well as your buttock and low back muscles. This exercise can improve standing and walking and help relieve low back pain. Do not perform this exercise if you have had a hip replacement.

1. Lie down on a firm, but not hard, surface, with knees raised.

2. Pull one knee to your chest until you feel a gentle stretch in your lower back, buttocks, and back of the thigh. The opposite leg should be slightly bent as shown.

3. Hold this position for 5 to 10 seconds and repeat 5 times. Then switch to the opposite side.

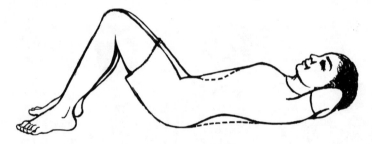

Fig. 13.6. Pelvic tilt: This is a classic exercise designed to help stabilize the pelvis, strengthen the abdominal muscles, and improve low back pain. Even if you don't have back pain, this is a good exercise to do.

1. Lie down on a firm, but not hard, surface, with knees raised.

2. Flatten your back by tightening your stomach and buttock muscles.

3. Hold this position for 5 seconds and repeat 5 times.

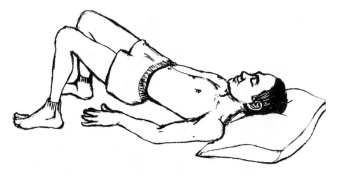

Fig. 13.7. Bridging: This exercise helps to stabilize the pelvis and low back as well as strengthen abdominal and low back muscles. 1. Lie down on a firm, but not hard, surface, with knees raised. 2. Focus on keeping your pelvis level and gently raise your buttocks from the floor. Keep your stomach muscles tight. 3. Gently lower your pelvis and repeat 5 times.

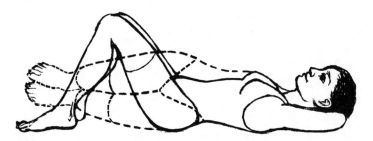

Fig. 13.8. Lower trunk stretch: This exercise helps to stretch low back, hip, and abdominal muscles. 1. Lie down on a firm, but not hard, surface, with knees raised. 2. Keeping your back flat and your feet together, rotate your knees to one side. 3. Hold this position for 5 seconds and then roll your knees to the opposite side for 5 seconds. Repeat 5 times.

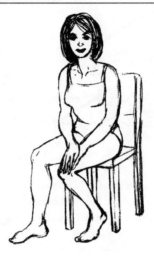

Fig. 13.9. Seated ankle stretch: This exercise improves the range of motion in the ankle by gently stretching the calf and heel cord. This can help with balance and walking. It can also decrease your overall mobility energy expenditure and reduce your risk of falling. Do not do this exercise if you have had an ankle fusion.
1. In a seated position, bend your knee and gently push to feel a stretch in your calf. Your heel should be off the floor.
2. Hold for 10 seconds. Repeat 5 times and switch sides.

Passive exercises, also called *passive stretches* or *passive range of motion exercises,* have been advocated by some as the only exercises appropriate for polio survivors—primarily because passive exercises are always nonfatiguing (someone else is doing the work). This advice is misguided; it should be interpreted as meaning that passive exercises may be quite helpful and are certainly nonfatiguing, but are usually not the only exercises polio survivors can do safely.

EXERCISING TO IMPROVE ENDURANCE

This type of exercising generally refers to *cardiovascular conditioning* or *aerobic exercise.* In a nutshell, cardiovascular fitness is the ability

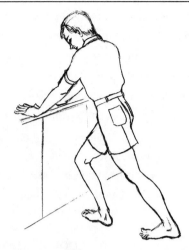

Fig. 13.10. Standing ankle stretch. This exercise is similar to 13.9 but is done in a standing position. Again, do not do this exercise if you have had an ankle fusion.
1. In a standing position, lean your hands against a wall or counter.
2. Keep your back leg straight with your heel on the floor.
3. Lean into the wall or counter until you feel a gentle stretch in your calf.
4. Hold for 10 seconds. Repeat 5 times and switch sides.

of the heart and blood vessels to work efficiently in order to supply the rest of the body with oxygen and other essential nutrients. The terms *cardiovascular conditioning, heart conditioning,* and *aerobic conditioning* may be used interchangeably to describe exercises that improve endurance.

The goal of a cardiovascular exercise regimen is to keep the heart rate at an elevated level for a given period. The Surgeon General advises "people of all ages to include a minimum of thirty minutes of physical activity of moderate intensity (such as brisk walking) on most, if not all, days of the week."[5] Although for the most part this is good advice, it may be excessive for some polio survivors.

John Wilson is a seventy-year-old polio survivor who recently underwent open-heart surgery. Afterward he noticed that he was feeling very tired and deconditioned. Even simple household chores fatigued him and he would become short of breath. John's cardiologist recommended that he start an exercise program to improve his endurance and cardiovascular fitness, and referred him to our polio clinic. After John underwent an evaluation, he started supervised physical therapy in order to develop an exercise program that would benefit him. The exercises that John was taught focused on improving his endurance without causing severe fatigue. After three months John returned to his cardiologist and reported that he was feeling much more energetic and that he was no longer short of breath when he did chores at home.

EXERCISING TO IMPROVE COORDINATION

Coordination is the delicate balance when certain muscles are used to perform a task and all other muscles are inhibited. It is dependent on programming the brain to move the extremities in a precise manner. In order to program the brain in this way, however, one must do thousands of repetitions of a single movement or group of movements.

Therefore, exercises to improve coordination involve *repetition*. A specific task must be performed over and over again. Small children repeatedly practice new skills such as standing, crawling, walking, using a spoon, and drinking from a cup. Older children constantly work on mastery of new skills by improving their coordination. As adults, most of us have attained the skills that require intense practice, and exercising to improve coordination plays a less important role.

Most polio survivors probably do not need to focus extensively on exercising to improve coordination; however, under certain circumstances coordination may become a major part of one's exercise regimen. For instance, if a polio survivor wants to learn a new skill such as golfing or table tennis, practicing the skills required is essen-

Table 13.2 General exercise recommendations

Perform exercises in the morning, ideally after a shower when the muscles are
  most flexible.
Exercise slowly and smoothly. Do not bounce.
Do not cause pain; you should only feel a gentle stretch.
Do not hold your breath.
Do not exercise to the point of exhaustion.

Note: The illustrations in this chapter are meant to be a guide for gentle stretches to
improve flexibility. Check with your doctor if you are having problems with these exercises or would like exercises specifically for you.

tial. If a new brace or assistive device such as a cane is prescribed, a
polio survivor may need to practice a different mode of walking in
order to feel comfortable and safe.

Too often people start using a cane (or other assistive device)
without formal instruction. The results can be disastrous if they use
the cane on the wrong side or do not know how to advance their feet
or the cane correctly. An assistive device improperly used always
increases energy consumption and may lead to falls. Moreover, once
someone begins using an assistive device improperly, the gait patterns that are established become difficult to correct. Thus, although
most polio survivors do not require formal exercises to improve
coordination, there certainly are circumstances in which these exercises are critical.

Another time when exercises to improve coordination are important is after a medical event such as a stroke. A person may then
have difficulty doing tasks he or she previously took for granted.
In this situation, exercising to improve coordination may be very
helpful.

*Fred Samuels is a lively eighty-year-old polio survivor who has never
had significant polio-related problems. When he suffered a small stroke,
his doctors declared him "lucky" and told him that he had made a*

remarkable recovery. But ever since the stroke Fred has noticed that his balance is slightly precarious and he has fallen several times—once hitting his head hard enough to require stitches. Fred was evaluated at the polio clinic and underwent a course of physical therapy specifically designed to work on his balance and coordination. Several months later, Fred was back to his old self and was no longer falling.

The Benefits of Exercise

The benefits of exercising are both physical and psychological. Studies show that normal aging and loss of strength may be due largely to decreased activity and loss of interest in being physically active.[6] Many polio survivors believe that their daily activities are a sufficient physical workout and that additional exercises would be detrimental. In some cases this may be true. In many other cases, however, it may be prudent for a polio survivor to utilize pacing techniques in order not to become physically exhausted each day. Adding an appropriate exercise program specifically designed to improve strength, endurance, and heart conditioning may then be reasonable. The benefits of an exercise program should not be discounted in anyone. Fortunately, polio survivors can generally reap most (if not all) of the rewards of participating in a regular exercise routine. The following list of benefits is not meant to be exhaustive, but rather to highlight some of the positive effects of regular exercise.

1. The risk of serious heart disease may be decreased.

Polio survivors often ask why they should exercise at all if there is even the smallest risk of becoming weaker. One convincing reason is that exercise has been proven to lower the risk of heart disease, which is the *number one cause of death in both men and women in the United States.* Studies have shown that many polio survivors have poor cardiovascular conditioning,[7] due in part to their physical inactivity. Obviously, when considering exercise options, polio survivors need to take into account not only the possibility of new weakness but also the very serious risk of heart disease. Even low-intensity (nonfatiguing) exercise programs that are designed to improve cardiovascular conditioning can be helpful.

2. The likelihood of having a stroke (brain attack) is diminished.

According to statistics compiled by the American Heart Association, strokes or brain attacks are the leading cause of serious long-term disability in the United States, and the third leading cause of death (behind heart disease and cancer).[8] Exercising regularly can help decrease the likelihood of having a stroke.

3. The control of glucose (sugar) in diabetes can be improved.

An estimated 16 million persons in the United States have diabetes (both diagnosed and undiagnosed).[9] Unfortunately, the deleterious effects of diabetes on an individual's health are often underestimated. The disease has the potential to be extremely disabling and can even lead to premature death. Controlling blood sugar is essential and will help to limit the many serious problems associated with diabetes (vision loss, kidney failure, poor circulation, nerve injuries, and so on). Regardless of whether individuals have had polio in the past, if they have diabetes, exercise is one of the best ways to help control high glucose levels.

4. Some of the intellectual decline that is often considered "normal aging" can be slowed or prevented.

The effects of exercise in this regard have not been well studied; however, the topic is of great interest and speculation in medical research. Recent studies have had encouraging results, and the possibility exists that exercising regularly may help in this area.[10]

5. Prevention of osteoporosis may be augmented.

Osteoporosis is discussed in detail in Chapter 17; suffice it to say that exercise is a critical component of keeping bones thick, healthy, and strong.

6. Mood can be improved and depression possibly prevented.

The psychological benefits of exercise are many.[11] Some are physical, including the release in the body of chemicals such as endorphins, natural substances that help make us feel content and even happy. Exercising regularly helps to release these substances and can in turn ease symptoms of anxiety and/or depression. In addition, exercising regularly can help build confidence and improve physical limitations, which also can lead to feeling psychologically more peaceful.

7. Symptoms of musculoskeletal pain can be improved.

Studies have shown that people who exercise regularly have fewer complaints of pain than people who are more sedentary. Although certainly exercising can lead to injuries, those who do not exercise regularly are even more prone to injuries. Exercise seems to improve symptoms of musculoskeletal pain in the neck, low back, and shoulder—all common complaints of polio survivors. The likelihood of sustaining an injury is much less if one follows the steps given below (Starting an Exercise Program Safely).

8. Symptoms of fatigue will be diminished.

Exercise can relieve feelings of fatigue in several ways. True fatigue from muscle weakness can be improved by strengthening the muscles and increasing endurance, so that daily activities require less energy. Fatigue from depression can also be improved as the brain releases endorphins during exercise.

9. The risk of falling may be decreased.

Falls and subsequent further disability are topics so serious that Chapter 16 in its entirety is devoted to them. For now let us note that exercising regularly can improve balance, coordination, and strength—all necessary to help prevent falls. Exercising can also improve endurance, and this too will make falling less likely. Further, if a fall does occur, regular exercise lessens the risk of serious injury.

Starting an Exercise Program Safely

There is no substitute for starting an exercise program under the guidance of experts. The simple rules are as follows:

1. Consult a medical doctor who is an expert in treating polio survivors.
2. Tell the doctor about any other medical illnesses you have.
3. Tell the doctor about any aches and pains you have.
4. Undergo medical tests the doctor recommends.
5. Ask for a prescription to see a physical and/or occupational therapist who is skilled in designing exercise programs for polio survivors.
6. Start out slowly.
7. Report any symptoms of fatigue, pain, or feeling out of breath.
8. Pace yourself.

The topic of exercise in polio survivors is complex and often confusing. Balancing activity and rest is a constant struggle. Individuals are often justifiably fearful that overutilizing muscles that are already working hard to perform daily activities may result in permanent weakness. Yet exercise is a critical part of maintaining flexibility, strength, coordination, and endurance—all of which help promote quality of life and independence. Exercise is also important in decreasing the risk of serious injuries and illnesses. Exercising regularly has been shown to improve symptoms of musculoskeletal pain and is psychologically beneficial. Fortunately, most polio survivors are able to enjoy the benefits of exercise, as long as they have medical experts to guide them.

CHAPTER 14

Energy Conservation and Pacing

"My muscle power and endurance are as coins in my purse: I have only so many and they will buy only so much. I must live within my means, and to do this I have to economize: what do I want to buy and how can I buy it for the least possible cost?" These are the words of Hugh Gallagher, an award-winning writer and a polio quadriplegic who has remained self-sufficient for more than forty years. Describing how he manages his energy as he ages, Gallagher goes on to say: "Growing old with polio is a matter of economics: cost/benefit analysis. How much expenditure of limited energy for how much satisfaction. Minimize the exertion; maximize the pleasure."[1]

Gallagher's analogy is elegant and goes to the heart of the role of energy conservation and pacing, which are important parts of aging gracefully with polio. His philosophy essentially means that polio survivors should live their lives to the fullest and enjoy the things they love and are able to do; it also means that they should not constantly push themselves *because they can*. The concepts employed in energy conservation and pacing are designed to allow people to do the activities that are important to them and to limit those that do not necessarily provide enjoyment and may require large energy expenditures.

If you are a polio survivor, you may be tempted to skip this chapter. After all, you have probably spent your entire life making accommodations and trying to plan your activities around physical limitations. But even the most meticulous polio survivors can find ways to conserve energy and improve their quality of life.

Ten Steps to Having More Energy and Feeling Better

STEP 1. TAKE AN ENERGY INVENTORY.

One of the best ways to evaluate how you can *save* energy is to determine first how your energy is *spent.* Keeping a log of all activities over a given period is a fine way to look objectively at how frugally or frivolously your energy "coins" are being spent. In my clinic, polio survivors keep a log of activities in which they write down everything they do for three days (Table 14.1). They also document episodes of pain and fatigue and the time of day and the activities during which these occur. The occupational therapist in the clinic reviews the log with them and highlights each activity with different-colored markers according to the amount of energy needed to accomplish it. For instance, low-energy activities are highlighted in yellow, moderate-energy in green, and high-energy in red. The goal of the activity log is to have an abundance of yellow and green and a minimum of red highlighted activities. The amazing part of this process is seeing how individuals spend their energy and how simple lifestyle changes can move a high-energy activity into the low or moderate category. The occupational therapist's job is to advise people on how to do the things that are important to them while still conserving energy. An example of how the three-day log works is described below.

Table 14.1 Three-day log of activities

Step 1. Organize a notebook with space to write in for each hour of the day for three days.

Step 2. Record your activities each hour over the next three days.

Step 3. As you record your activities, also write down when you have pain or feel fatigued.

Step 4. After three days of recording your activities, take three different-colored highlighters and mark each hour of activity as low-energy, moderate energy, or high energy.

Step 5. Now analyze your three-day log. When do you feel the most pain? Is it when you are working without taking a break? When are you feeling tired? Can you plan for a rest period during the times you feel most fatigued?

Note: This log will differ for everyone and is simply a guide to help you analyze your activity level and correlate it with your pain and fatigue levels.

Mary Johnson is a fifty-five-year-old elementary-school secretary who contracted polio after the birth of her third child. During the initial episode, she had profound involvement of her pulmonary muscles and for weeks used an iron lung to breathe. Mary made a remarkable recovery, but thereafter had some arm weakness and shortness of breath owing to respiratory muscle weakness. Because she had difficulty breathing when she overexerted herself, Mary believed she was an expert at pacing and energy conservation and that nothing further could be done to help her get through her day. When Mary came for an evaluation, she was despondent and ready to quit the job she loved, saying, "I don't have the energy to make it through the day!" Reluctant at first to evaluate critically how she was spending her energy, Mary finally agreed to keep a three-day log of her activities. When she returned for a follow-up appointment, she exclaimed, "You won't believe this, but I got up from my desk more than fifty times in a single morning at work!" As part of the treatment protocol, an occupational therapist was sent to Mary's school to evaluate her workstation. After rearranging it and ordering some relatively inexpensive equipment (which the school purchased),

Mary was able to do her job without getting up more than a few times during the entire day! The three-day log also proved useful in other areas, and one year after instituting the pacing and energy conservation techniques she learned, Mary came in for another follow-up appointment and reported that she felt better than she had in ten years. She now easily makes it through her workday and revels in her newfound energy.

While not everyone will have such dramatic results, even a small improvement in energy level can significantly improve the quality of life. Diane Christy is a mother and professional educator. She has had a chronic illness since birth that has required her to make energy conservation a daily priority. Using her expertise in this area, she co-authored *Pacing Yourself.* Christy writes in the introduction, "Days become tapestries—intricate weavings of rests and planned activities, each with a special method or trick."[2]

STEP 2. TALK TO YOUR DOCTOR.

Many of the ways in which energy is dramatically consumed result from readily treatable medical conditions. For example, untreated injuries or diseases such as arthritis make it more difficult to move around with ease. Essentially any medical condition may sap one's energy. The key to stopping the energy drain is to have these problems treated. Keep in mind that the process may be ongoing (particularly in chronic conditions such as arthritis) and you may need to visit the doctor regularly for "fine-tuning." The burden of moving about with pain causes much more than physical discomfort—it wastes precious energy stores! Think of pain as being a voice that says, "Go to the doctor and get some help in order to conserve energy."

Energy is also wasted when polio survivors get weaker and their walking changes. Any changes in mobility in general (such as transfers) will cause an increase in energy utilization. In order to minimize energy expenditures, a polio doctor can recommend ways to make walking or moving about easier—perhaps trying lightweight braces or using a motorized scooter or wheelchair. Many individuals are resistant to changing the way they get around. I always encourage people to consider how valuable it is to them to be able to move with ease and conserve energy. I ask them, "If moving around more easily would allow you to do things that are meaningful to you and would improve your quality of life, would you consider alternative ways to be mobile?" Most polio survivors want to find easier and less taxing ways of moving about. Those who do not simply choose to use a more significant portion of their energy coins for mobility purposes. There is no right or wrong way. You need to define what is meaningful to you and how you are going to live your life to the fullest.

STEP 3. EVALUATE YOUR SLEEP HABITS.

One of the most obvious reasons people complain of low energy is that they fail to get enough sleep, or the right kind of sleep. If you answer any of the following questions affirmatively, you may want to consult with your doctor about a possible sleep disorder.

1. Do you have difficulty falling asleep?
2. Do you have difficulty staying asleep?
3. Do you snore?
4. Do you have repeated nightmares?
5. Do you have difficulty breathing either during the day or at night?
6. Is your sleep restless?
7. Do you wake in the morning and still feel tired?

Problems with sleep may be due to respiratory issues related to having had polio, or they may result from a variety of other medical conditions such as depression, anxiety, or sleep apnea. Sometimes sleep habits can be improved by simple lifestyle changes such as avoiding caffeine late in the day. Alcohol, although a sedative, may contribute to fatigue and inefficient sleep habits.

STEP 4. CONSIDER LOSING WEIGHT.

This is a difficult step, and there is no simple prescription. Chapter 15 is devoted to nutrition and weight management, but the truth is that different things work for different people. For polio survivors who have limited ability to exercise, losing weight sometimes requires a Herculean effort. Unfortunately, the bottom line is that excess weight creates a constant drain on your body's energy resources. If you want to know the extent of the drain, try this exercise. Calculate how many pounds of extra weight you are currently carrying. Then take household items that weigh approximately the same amount and try to carry them around for an entire day. Chances are that after a few minutes you will realize that the effort required to do this for an entire day is extraordinary. Maybe this exercise will give you the impetus you need to lose weight. Extra weight means less energy to do the things you enjoy; *lots* of extra weight means lots less energy to do the things you enjoy.

STEP 5. GET ORGANIZED.

Disorganization is a terrible waste of precious energy. Organizing physical space, as well as organizing time spent on activities during the day, is critical to conserving energy. Start with the physical space: get rid of clutter. If an item has not been used in the past year, consider giving it to someone who can use it or throw it away. A home and office that are clutter free will allow easy access to the essentials. Equally important is organizing what remains after the clutter is cleared.

Next, organize the day by planning ahead. Group errands by geographic location. Make lists for the grocery store, the mall, wherever you need to go. Use available delivery services for groceries, dry cleaning, and pharmacy. Use the telephone to comparison shop. The Internet provides wonderful opportunities to shop from home. Formally writing down errands in order of priority will allow you to select only those that are necessary or particularly enjoyable. It will also enable you to consider other ways of getting these things done (perhaps asking a friend to help or ordering by telephone). Although becoming more organized does take some initial input of energy, the long-term cost savings in energy coins is well worth it!

Kay Miller is a sixty-year-old survivor of bulbar polio who admits she is thoroughly disorganized. She hates to make lists and thinks that becoming organized is more work than it is worth. Kay confided to me one day that her friends have nicknamed her Kay-os (chaos) because she is so disorganized. When I ultimately convinced her to make a few minor changes in order to organize her daily activities, she was surprised at how much more energy she had at the end of the day.

STEP 6. SIMPLIFY.

Simplifying daily routines and chores can add hours to the day and markedly save on energy costs. Persons with polio are not the only ones who need to strive to make their lives simpler. The vast majority of popular magazines routinely contain time-saving and energy-saving techniques. Even geniuses look for ways to conserve energy. According to Gerald Holton, a professor of physics at Harvard University, it is well known that Albert Einstein was "parsimonious" in his approach to both physics and his personal life. One of the many ways in which Einstein simplified his life was by owning several identical sets of clothing. That way he never had to stop and consider what to wear each day.

Einstein was a brilliant but quirky man, and not everyone would embrace his energy-conserving ideas. However, there are many easy ways to simplify daily routines in order to save energy. For example, make enough dinner to have leftovers for the next night; choose a simple wardrobe without unnecessary accessories, buttons, or snaps; shave every other or every third day; have your mail and newspapers delivered to the door rather than left at the street level; and order groceries by phone, fax, or computer and have them delivered. The appendix to this chapter gives a more complete list of ways to conserve energy.

STEP 7. TALK TO FAMILY AND FRIENDS.

Often it is not easy for persons with a history of polio to ask for help or let family and friends know that things are becoming more difficult. Conditioned to be independent and uncomplaining, polio survivors sometimes find it hard to express thoughts that may leave them feeling vulnerable. But family and friends are vital members of our support structures, and they need to understand what is happening so that they can continue to be supportive. A frank conversation is a reasonable way to start. Let people know what is happening and how they can be of help. Then when it is time, let them help!

Family members or friends who are truly supportive will appreciate hearing how they can help. Moreover, not having an honest conversation may lead to misunderstanding. A partner may feel increasingly burdened with doing more than his or her share of the household chores, or may be frightened watching the loved one struggle to maintain the status quo. Helping that person understand the changes that are occurring will give reassurance. Ultimately, if a polio survivor explains what is happening and why it is important to conserve energy, friends and family are likely to be understanding and supportive.

STEP 8. PLAN REST PERIODS.

Resting periodically is not the same as planning rest periods. Actually scheduling rest periods during the day is a surefire way to reenergize. Unscheduled rest periods may be missed altogether or may not occur until a polio survivor is thoroughly exhausted. Many have described their fatigue by saying, for instance, "I just seem to hit a wall," or "A dark curtain comes down and I can no longer function." Scheduling rest periods during the day can help avoid getting to the "point of no return," when fatigue becomes completely disabling. Keep in mind that planning a rest period does not necessarily mean taking a nap, which in many instances is not feasible. Mary Johnson, as an example, arranged to lie down in the teacher's lounge and read a book for twenty minutes twice a day. These were her scheduled breaks, which she had traditionally taken when the teachers took theirs. Instead of having a cup of coffee and talking to her colleagues, Mary found it much more relaxing to take her breaks separately and to read a book or simply rest on the couch. Other ways to rejuvenate oneself include deep breathing exercises, yoga, and listening to classical music (see Table 14.2 for other examples).

Plan rest periods also in a more elaborate manner by taking vacations from your daily routine. Patients often ask me whether it would help them to have more energy if they worked fewer hours. My standard suggestion is that they find out for themselves via a reduced-hours trial by using some of their vacation time. If you think that you are working too hard (either at home or at work), then take a vacation or reduce your schedule and see if that helps. If it does, you have your answer.

Table 14.2   Ways to relax without sleeping

Listen to music.
Listen to relaxation tapes.
Watch television.
Read a book or magazine.
Meditate and/or pray.
Sit down and talk to someone in person or on the phone.
Perform deep breathing and relaxation exercises.
Play a game on the computer or with a friend.
Sit in your favorite chair with a warm drink (decaffeinated and nonalcoholic is
    best).
Lie down and take time to reflect.
Go for a scenic drive.

Note: This is not meant to be a complete list, but rather to suggest ways to take a break
during the day.

STEP 9. FOLLOW THE WEATHER REPORTS.

Inclement weather can take its toll on anyone's energy level. Either
extreme of barometric pressure is taxing. Obviously no one can alter
weather patterns, but being aware of the forecast can be useful in
conserving energy. During periods of extreme heat, high humidity,
rain, or snow, plan to do only the essentials. When the weather
improves, postponed errands and chores can be done more easily.

Another reason to avoid the energy drain that occurs during
poor weather is that this is when people are vulnerable to falling and
getting injured. Falls are particularly likely in cold weather, when the
ground is slick from rain or snow. Hot days can be draining and
energy levels very low. Fatigue during warm weather can also lead to
overuse of the muscles and potential falls.

But staying indoors on very hot or very cold days is not enough:
the indoor temperature must be maintained at a comfortable setting. Saving money on heating or air-conditioning expenses is apt to
take its toll on physical stamina. The real money you save may not

be as valuable to you as the energy coins that are wasted trying to maintain your body temperature in an uncomfortable indoor climate.

STEP 10. RECOGNIZE SIGNS OF DEPRESSION AND
ISOLATION.

Commonly, individuals with ongoing medical problems feel frustrated, isolated, and even depressed. Although this is a natural response, recognizing symptoms of depression is critical in any chronic illness, and particularly in PPS. The fatigue caused by depression may be confused with the fatigue caused by PPS. Many polio survivors have learned to their chagrin that the unhappiness, pain, and fatigue they experience is caused by a chronic depression of which they were unaware. Few persons, no matter how perceptive, can diagnose their own depression.

Since depression is treatable and often curable (particularly the situational depressions that occur owing to a change in health, as is possible with PPS), it is critical to have a medical doctor diagnose and treat the depression along with the PPS. Treating one or the other alone is rarely effective. Many polio survivors think that asking for help with depression is a sign of weakness or that it is simply another way in which their body has "let them down." It becomes a vicious cycle: "If only I could get around better and do more, I wouldn't feel so sad." Conversely, "If only I didn't feel so sad, I would have more energy to get around and do more."

Don Goldenberg is a rheumatologist who has battled chronic illness for much of his adult life. In his book *Chronic Illness and Uncertainty,* he describes how he would avoid sitting in the waiting room of his psychiatrist's office and instead hide in his car until it was time for his appointment. In an honest and poignant chapter on depression and how it relates to chronic illness, he discusses his own

Table 14.3   Symptoms of depression

Losing interest in usual activities and pastimes
Feeling irritable
Crying frequently
Feeling sad
Feeling hopeless
Having poor appetite or significant weight loss
Having increased appetite or significant weight gain
Sleeping poorly
Sleeping too much
Feeling agitated or restless
Feeling fatigued (particularly in the morning when usually refreshed after a
     night's rest)
Having difficulty concentrating
Having difficulty making decisions
Feeling self-critical
Feeling excessively guilty
Feeling worthless
Having recurrent thoughts of dying or suicidal thoughts

---

experience and its effect on his health. "The medically sophisticated person knows that, however enlightened his or her own view of depression and psychiatry, many people will not understand. Our society's continuing failure to accept mood disturbances as 'legitimate' illness forces patients to feel embarrassed. It often causes them to deny their depression and avoid treatment that could help them. They must bear loss of self-esteem, along with their depression. They feel frail or inadequate, as I did, and guilty for 'bringing this on myself.' I now believe that my recurrent bouts of fatigue were caused or at least exacerbated by unrecognized long-standing depression and anxiety."[3]

Pacing and energy-conservation techniques are designed to enable polio survivors to improve their quality of life. Taken to the extreme (that is, conserving energy at all times regardless of the activity) can be very isolating. The more isolated someone feels, the more

Table 14.4 Symptoms of anxiety

Feeling tense or nervous
Feeling jittery or jumpy
Having difficulty relaxing
Feeling fatigued
Having muscle ache
Feeling restless
Feeling apprehensive
Feeling fearful or anticipating misfortune
Feeling sweaty or having clammy hands
Feeling chest palpitations or heart racing
Having a stomachache
Feeling light-headed or dizzy
Having difficulty sleeping
Feeling "on edge"
Feeling terrified without apparent reason
Anticipating impending doom
Feeling short of breath
Experiencing a choking or smothering sensation
Feeling faint
Trembling or shaking

---

likely he or she will become depressed, and vice versa. Therefore, energy-conservation techniques should always be utilized in moderation, with the goal of *improving the quality of life.* On the other hand, failing to utilize energy-conservation and pacing techniques can also lead to isolation and depression, as the individual feels more tired and less able to participate in the activities that give pleasure. Striking an appropriate balance between activity and rest is essential.

Regardless of the energy techniques used, a person who is feeling sad, anxious, or depressed may also be feeling fatigued. The fatigue may be due to difficulty sleeping at night or it may be a symptom of a medical condition such as depression or an anxiety disorder. (Tables 14.3 and 14.4 describe symptoms associated with these medical conditions.) Any symptoms that may indicate a mood disorder (depression, anxiety, and so forth) should be discussed with a medical doctor. A physician experienced in treating polio survivors generally can determine which symptoms may be related to previous polio and which may indicate a different diagnosis. Once the cause of the symptoms is determined, the doctor can prescribe appropriate treatment and recommend other health-care providers who may be helpful.

Energy conservation and pacing are critical to aging gracefully with polio. To recall Gallagher's analogy, the goals of energy conservation and pacing are not to be miserly with one's energy coins, but rather to spend them wisely in order to improve one's quality of life.

Appendix
Pacing and Energy-Conservation Techniques

General

Learn to set priorities and eliminate unnecessary tasks.
Plan ahead and avoid last-minute changes and rushing.
Plan activities to avoid unnecessary walking and stair climbing.
Ask for assistance when you need or want it.

Home

GENERAL

Ask the mail and newspaper delivery persons to drop off these items at your door.
Create a paper management center to pay bills, organize coupons, etc.
On a conveniently located bulletin board, post important dates, menus for food delivery services, and phone numbers.
Use commercial organizers to save space and improve organization.

BATHING

Sit in the bath or shower (use a nonskid tub bench or shower chair).
Keep all bathing products on a shelf within easy reach.
Use shampoo with built-in conditioner, to save a step.

DRESSING

Sit for dressing.

Select simple clothing without a lot of buttons, snaps, or hooks.

Buy sturdy but lightweight shoes.

Wear simple shoes with laces, straps, or buckles.

Sit down and use a long-handled shoehorn to put on shoes.

GROOMING

Sit for grooming.

Lay out grooming products and makeup in the order you want to use them.

Use an electric toothbrush.

Use multipurpose products to save steps (e.g., moisturizer with sunscreen).

Use an overhead hair dryer rather than a hand-held blow dryer.

GROCERY SHOPPING

Order groceries by phone, fax, or computer and have them delivered.

Always use a grocery list and develop a standard shopping list to avoid writing a new one each time.

Ask that perishables be bagged separately so all groceries don't have to be put away at once.

Use a wheeled cart to bring groceries that are not delivered from the car to the house.

Buy smaller cartons and packages to avoid excessive lifting (e.g., buy a quart or half-gallon of milk rather than a gallon).

Ask friends or neighbors to pick up extra items when they go shopping.

Shop consistently in a store you know well, to find items easily.

Check the supermarket directory to avoid hunting for obscure items.

COOKING

Sit down to prepare meals.

Keep items most frequently used within easy reach.

Slide or roll heavy items toward you before lifting them.

Prepare extra food so that you have leftovers for the next day.

Use prepared foods and mixes whenever possible.

Place refrigerated items most often used at a level to avoid reaching and bending.

Wear an apron with pockets in order to carry things more easily.

Use a wheeled cart to bring items from the refrigerator to the stove or table where they are needed.

Use paper plates and napkins and plastic utensils for easy cleanup.

Use wide-handled cooking utensils (which require less strength to grip) for chopping vegetables, etc.

Use an electric blender for mixing and chopping.

Use an electric can opener.

Use a jar opener.

Instead of using the oven (which requires a lot of bending and reaching), use a table-size toaster oven, crock-pot, or electric skillet.

Line cooking pans with foil and discard when finished to avoid messy cleanup.

Use the front burners on the stove to avoid excessive reaching.

Use a timer to avoid getting up and down to check whether the meal is done.

Soak dishes first to avoid scrubbing.

Let dishes air dry.

Use a dishwasher if possible.

CLEANING

If possible, hire someone to clean your home regularly.

Decorate your home simply to avoid unnecessary dusting around small decorative items.

Use a long-handled duster.

Use a long-handled dust pan to avoid stooping when sweeping the floor.

Use a squeegee mop or long-handled sponge to wipe down the shower or bath.

Use a wheeled cart to take out the trash.

Avoid buying economy-size cleaning products; stick with smaller sizes that are more manageable.

Use a self-propelled vacuum cleaner.

LAUNDRY

Buy permanent-press clothing to avoid unnecessary ironing.

Use a dry cleaning service that delivers to your home.

Avoid lifting boxes of detergent or bleach; instead, use a cup or measuring utensil to dispense what you need.

Use multipurpose laundry products such as detergents with bleach.

Do small laundry loads to avoid excessive lifting and carrying.

Use a wheeled cart or hamper on casters if you live in a single-level home.

Use a high-quality, lightweight travel iron for all your ironing.

Don't iron items such as sheets, towels, pajamas, etc.

Use a rubber plunger for hand washables to prevent finger and hand overuse.

Wash as many hand washables as feasible in the machine, using delicate cycle and special detergent.

Sit down when ironing (this can be done at the kitchen table with a towel protecting the table).

Place a table in the laundry area from which clothes can be loaded and unloaded from a top-loading washer or dryer.

YARDWORK

Keep your yard simple and avoid excessive gardening.

Ask a friend or hire someone to mow your lawn and trim your hedges.

Ask a friend or hire someone to plow your driveway and shovel your walkway in winter.

Office

Sit in a chair with firm back and arm supports.

Keep papers and documents at eye level without holding them, by using a copy stand or document holder.

Consider using a track ball instead of a mouse for your computer.

Be sure your arms are supported when writing or keyboarding at your workstation (special forearm rests are available commercially).

Plan your workstation so as to avoid getting up excessively or constantly having to reach for items.

Consider using voice-activated software for your computer, rather than typing.

Leisure

Use a book stand or copy stand to read books, magazines, and other documents.

Use a speaker phone or telephone headset to avoid holding the phone receiver.

Use a remote control to change channels on the television or stations on the radio.

Avoid low chairs.

Errands

Consider using a left-foot gas pedal or hand controls for your car.

Use cruise control for long distances.

Use an automatic garage door opener.

Obtain a handicapped license plate or placard and routinely use parking spaces designated for persons with disabilities.

Use a manual wheelchair only when someone else is doing the pushing.

Use a motorized scooter or wheelchair, particularly in malls, airports, amusement parks, etc.

Use a pack that attaches around your waist (fanny pack) to carry personal items.

If you need to carry a purse or briefcase, make it as light as possible and use a shoulder strap.

Combine errands to avoid extra trips.

Use a car phone and call ahead to see if your order is ready; ask if someone is available to bring it to your car.

Call ahead for appointments in order to limit the amount of time you have to wait.

Call ahead and find out if the place you are going is accessible (e.g., are there stairs to climb?).

Ask friends and family when they are going to the post office, etc. and arrange to have them drop off your packages or help you with errands.

Schedule appointments either first thing in the morning or right after lunch, to avoid waiting.

Ask for prescriptions to be called in to the pharmacy by someone at the doctor's office.

Travel

When taking longer trips, use a standard packing list.

Pack a small bag with just the essentials.

Use luggage with wheels and arrange for a porter whenever possible.

If your flight is canceled, use a pay phone at the airport to arrange for a new flight instead of standing in a long line at the counter.

CHAPTER 15

Nutrition and Weight

Attempting to write a chapter that addresses nutrition and weight issues while providing surefire ways to stay trim and fit is a recipe for failure. No chapter (or even book) can reveal the "secrets" of proper nutrition and ideal weight management, in part because dietary recommendations change frequently as medical science learns more about how food affects health and disease. Even more important is that individuals often require advice that is more specific than generic, in order to take into account their health history, dietary preferences, exercise restrictions, weight fluctuations, and target weight.

Nevertheless, the subjects of diet, nutrition, and weight are so crucial that I would be remiss to ignore them altogether in this book. I hope this chapter will at least help polio survivors to gain perspective on how these issues contribute to health and well-being, or in some cases to further disability and even death.

Weight and Its Relationship to Disease and Disability

The effects of increased body fat, particularly (but not exclusively) in the middle of the body, need to be considered in everyone. Obesity is associated with a host of serious medical conditions and increased risk of death. It can result in increased risk of high blood pressure (which can lead to stroke), heart disease, diabetes, and even certain types of cancer. Individuals who are overweight are also likely to have osteoarthritis of the joints, with pain and decreased mobility. Obesity can also affect respiratory function and can greatly exacerbate breathing problems in polio survivors. The unfortunate social stigma associated with weight issues may cause individuals to suffer psychologically—regardless of how much they weigh.

For polio survivors, carrying around even a few extra pounds requires energy and muscle power that may make mobility increasingly difficult and in some instances contribute to further weakness. Excess weight may also impact an individual's balance and lead to falls, with subsequent serious injury and disability. In polio survivors suffering from fatigue, the burden of extra weight may worsen their symptoms.

In order to determine how *much* extra weight can impact your balance, mobility, fatigue, or pain level, try the following exercise. Think of how much weight you would need to lose in order to be at your ideal weight. (Remember that polio survivors cannot always use standardized charts as their criteria, since paralysis and atrophy of the muscles decrease overall weight.) Visualize that number as a slab of beef that you would purchase at the store. How much effort would it require for you to carry that slab of beef for an entire day? At the end of the day when you could set it down, would it be a relief? Would you feel less pain? Less fatigue? Would you be able to move more easily?

When I counsel polio survivors on weight loss, I try to get them to imagine how getting rid of extra weight might make them more agile and energetic. Because losing weight can be difficult and can take considerable time, I encourage them to picture what it would be like to shed even one or two pounds. To a body that is working at its maximal capacity, eliminating even a small load can be a tremendous relief.

While most polio survivors struggle with being overweight, some are actually underweight. This, too, can lead to a host of problems including malnutrition, frailty, bone loss, and lack of energy. Regardless of whether someone is overweight or underweight, seeking professional guidance is vital—particularly in polio survivors, who are at risk for significant further disability.

The options for weight management may include investigative tests to rule out medical conditions that can cause weight gain or loss. Your doctor may opt to refer you to another physician or health-care provider. In my practice, I work closely with a nutritionist who understands the exercise limitations of polio survivors; together we counsel individuals on how to gradually make dietary changes that will help them to manage their weight as they age.

Diet and Nutrition and Their Impact on Physical Health

Regardless of how much someone weighs, a healthy, balanced diet is essential to maintaining physical health and well-being. The details of a balanced diet, although beyond the scope of this book, can be found in any of the reputable books on diet and nutrition and are important for polio survivors to consider. Here are a few general guidelines:

1. Eat small portions that are low in fat and contain adequate protein and other nutrients.
2. Have healthy midmorning and midafternoon snacks to keep your energy level high.
3. Avoid eating at night after dinner.
4. Avoid taking excessive vitamins and other nutritional supplements unless recommended by your doctor.
5. Avoid tobacco in any form.

6. Limit alcohol intake as much as possible. Alcohol adds unnecessary calories, increases symptoms of fatigue, decreases balance, and in excess amounts can cause a number of serious medical conditions.

7. Check with your doctor regarding any nutritional deficiencies prior to starting a weight-loss or weight-gain program.

Weight management and proper nutrition are essential in order to age gracefully with polio. Unfortunately, no magic pill or potion will obviate the need to work diligently at optimizing weight and nutritional status. Many polio survivors have the burden of not being able to manage their weight, even in part, through aggressive exercise. Nevertheless, staying trim and eating nutritiously will undoubtedly help to prevent further disability in polio survivors as they age.

CHAPTER 16

Preventing Falls and Further Disability

Falling is perhaps the single most disabling event that can occur in an individual with a history of paralytic polio. The statistics in the general population on falls and subsequent disability are staggering. Accidents are the sixth leading cause of death in persons over sixty-five years of age, and falls account for two-thirds of these deaths.[1] Approximately 30 percent of persons over the age of sixty-five and more than 50 percent of those over age eighty who are living independently will experience at least one fall each year.[2] The annual number of hip fractures in the United States is 250,000. For persons who sustain a hip fracture, the mortality rate the following year is between 15 and 20 percent.[3] Moreover, someone who repeatedly falls is extremely likely to enter a nursing home. The fear of falling while alone may lead to a self-imposed reduction in physical activity and negatively impact one's quality of life.[4]

For a number of reasons, polio survivors are at even greater risk than the general population of falling and sustaining a serious injury. First, many have had a lifetime of falling periodically and consider themselves "experts in the art of falling." Perhaps because they have not been injured in the past, or perhaps because they fail to realize that most falls are preventable, some polio survivors accept falls as a way of life. Second, as polio survivors age, they may experience increasing weakness and difficulty with balance and coordination. As these issues become relevant, many polio survivors simply start using an assistive device (cane, crutch, walker), without any formal training. The device may be too large or too small, may be used incorrectly, or may not even be the ideal solution. Third, many polio survivors have other medical problems that, left untreated, may cause further disability and the propensity to fall. For example, a tendinitis of the rotator cuff muscles in the shoulder can make transfers more difficult and walking with an assistive device more precarious. This injury is treatable and potentially curable, and should be addressed by a medical doctor. Fourth, because of the paralysis from the initial polio, the bones surrounding the fully or partially paralyzed muscles are almost always thinner and more fragile than the bones surrounded by unaffected muscles. These bones, called osteopenic or osteoporotic, are highly susceptible to fracture when a fall occurs. In some cases the bones are so thin that they actually fracture first and then the fall occurs. Fifth, polio survivors who have upper-extremity weakness lack the ability to protect themselves effectively with their arms once they lose their balance. The result is often an essentially unprotected fall in which the blow to the body is substantial. Last, polio survivors are susceptible to all of the same risk factors for falling (described below) as the general population. For all of these reasons, polio survivors are at an enormously increased risk for falling and sustaining a serious injury. Every attempt should be made to mitigate the number of falls.

Prevention of Falls

The vast majority of falls (more than 80 percent) are preventable occurrences. While there are instances when an individual falls unavoidably, these falls are not typical of most that occur. In fact, experts who study falls rarely categorize falls as accidental, but rather choose to call them preventable occurrences. In order to understand how falls can be prevented, it is necessary to first understand how they occur.

All falls occur because of either intrinsic or extrinsic risk factors (Table 16.1).[5] Intrinsic factors are those that affect how one's body works. Risk factors for falling due to an intrinsic cause include poor balance, weakness, effect of medications, and poor eyesight or hearing. Extrinsic factors are environmentally related and include uneven walking surfaces, poor weather conditions, and use of heavy or broken braces.

Intrinsic and extrinsic factors may play a simultaneous role. Studies reveal that as many as 35 percent of all falls resulting in injury occur in the home in familiar surroundings.[6] One reason, obviously, is that the home is where people spend most of their time. But people also are probably less cautious in a familiar environment. There may be other reasons as well. As individuals age, they may have more difficulty cleaning and maintaining their homes. Hazards may accumulate, such as soap scum on the tub or shower floor, items left unattended on the floor, poor lighting due to burned-out bulbs, and the like. The opposite may also be true: overzealous cleaning and waxing of floors may leave them wet and slippery, making falls more likely. Pets may pose a threat as they scurry underfoot or lie quietly on the floor. Many people discount minor "trips and slips" at home, not realizing that these may lead to a fall and a serious injury. One study noted that "trips and slips were the most prevalent causes of falls," accounting for nearly 60 percent.[7] The majority of these trips and slips result from extrinsic factors and are easily avoided by making the home environment safer.

Intrinsic factors are also involved in the numbers of falls occurring at home. Home is where individuals generally take their medications, and these may affect alertness and balance. Home is also

Table 16.1 Intrinsic and extrinsic risk factors for falls

Intrinsic risk factors:
Poor vision
Poor hearing
Blood pressure abnormalities
Anemia
Irregular heart rate
Medication effects
Poor balance
Foot problems
Weakness
Inflexibility
Pain
Infections (especially those that cause fever)
Psychological disturbances (e.g., depression, grief)
Fatigue
Dizziness
Frequent urination (especially at night)

Extrinsic risk factors:
Poor lighting
Slippery tub or shower floor
Lack of grab bars in bathroom
Uneven or slick floor surfaces
Clutter
Throw rugs
Raised doorjambs
Exposed extension cords
Stairs without secure railings
Furniture that is too low or too high
Holding onto furniture while moving about
Furniture without sturdy arm supports
Shelves that are too low or too high
Improper footwear
Old, heavy, or broken braces
Improper assistive devices (e.g., canes, crutches, walkers)
Inclement weather conditions
Crowded places that increase the likelihood of getting bumped or pushed

where individuals often indulge in alcoholic beverages, which invariably affect balance and sometimes alertness—even one or two drinks! At home, people are more likely to let down their guard, perhaps leaving their glasses on a table and moving about with impaired vision, or propping their cane against a table rather than using it (a double hazard, because they have left the cane in a place where they may potentially trip on it!).

During the night, many individuals get up to go to the bathroom, and that can be hazardous. Still somewhat sedated, they are more likely to fall when they get up quickly in the dark and move about. Further complicating this nighttime ritual is the dilemma of whether to bother putting on cumbersome shoes and braces.

Yet the home is not the only place where falls occur. They are also a potential threat out in the community or in unfamiliar surroundings. Certainly falls are more likely to occur in inclement weather, when the ground is slippery or icy. They may also occur if accessibility is a problem. For example, an individual may experience an unusual level of fatigue that leads to a fall shortly after climbing a set of stairs when an elevator is not available.[8] Or this individual may trip and fall on the stairs themselves if there is no railing. Invariably, being out in the community involves some hazards. Planning ahead and stopping for rest periods are essential in order to avoid becoming overly tired and risking a fall when away from home.

Injuries from Falls

Many types of injuries can occur after a fall, and while some are rather trivial, others may be life threatening or result in permanent disability (Table 16.2).[9] Most falls result in either no injury or in minor soft-tissue injuries such as bruises and abrasions. More serious injuries include fractures of the extremities and the vertebrae in the spine. One of the most serious consequences of a fall is internal

Table 16.2 Common injuries from falls

Soft tissue (e.g., bruises, abrasions)
Bony fractures (hip, forearm, and vertebral are the most common)
Head injuries (concussions and internal bleeding are the most common)
Lacerations (often requiring stitches)
Muscle, ligament, and tendon injuries (e.g., neck strain, ankle sprain)
Joint and cartilage injuries (e.g., torn cartilage or meniscus in the knee)

---

bleeding, which may occur when a fall results in hitting the head and the resulting injury to the small blood vessels around the brain. Frequently called subdural hematoma, this type of trauma can result in serious brain injury or death.

Another well-known phenomenon after someone has fallen is that they become fearful of having another fall. This fear can be psychologically disabling and can cause social isolation leading to depression. While the fear of falling is not an injury per se, it may be the most disabling consequence of a fall. For a variety of reasons, polio survivors are at a much higher risk for having multiple falls and for sustaining serious injury than age-matched individuals who have not had polio.

Anyone with paralysis is almost certain to have thinning of the bones owing to a lack of the muscular contraction that keeps bones thick and strong. A history of polio combined with normal aging often leads to unusually fragile bones that may easily break—sometimes without any trauma at all! More often, bone fractures occur in polio survivors as the result of falls. The topic of how to keep healthy bones is so important that I devote Chapter 17 in its entirety to osteoporosis.

Myths about Falling

Many of the myths about falls, when believed and perpetuated, lead to more falls and subsequently to the potential for further disability. Dispelling these myths is essential to protection from a serious injury.

MYTH 1. FALLS ARE ACCIDENTAL AND THEREFORE CANNOT BE PREDICTED OR PREVENTED.

This is absolutely false. Most falls are quite predictable and can be prevented with proper attention to intrinsic and extrinsic risk factors.

John Melon is a forty-five-year-old, highly successful businessman who owns and manages multiple restaurants in several towns. After his initial polio at age four, John had multiple surgeries on his right leg and was able to walk without any braces or assistive devices. When he first came to see me, he was simply scouting out experts who treated polio patients. John denied having any of the symptoms of PPS; however, when asked about falls, he nonchalantly reported falling several times each month. He was initially surprised at how persistently I pursued the issue of falls with him. For John, falling was a way of life. Even more disturbing was that on his second visit, after discussing with his wife how often he falls, John reported that he had underestimated the frequency and confided that he actually falls several times each week! After a great deal of counseling, John agreed that it was only a matter of time before he incurred a serious injury that would cause him further disability (he already limped, and not unexpectedly his balance was precarious). Initially opposed to any type of bracing, John reluctantly agreed to try a sleek and lightweight ankle-foot orthosis (short leg brace), which was dyed black to make it less noticeable. In the course of several visits with the physical therapist, John learned how to walk with his new brace and how to change his home and work environments to decrease the risk of falling. Three years later, at his annual follow-up appointment, John reported that he had not fallen since his earliest visit.

The example above illustrates several points. First, simply increasing someone's awareness that falling is dangerous can prevent falls. Second, evaluation of bracing needs by a medical expert is important. Third, gait training and help with balance and coordination in a formal physical therapy setting can be extremely beneficial. Fourth, an evaluation of the home and office environments is ideal. Last, falls should not be considered accidental, but instead predictable and preventable.

MYTH 2. AN OCCASIONAL FALL IS EXPECTED AND ACCEPTABLE.

In *no* circumstances is falling acceptable. Theoretically not every fall can be prevented, but an attempt should be made to prevent all falls. Even if an individual only falls once, he or she may sustain a serious and potentially life-threatening injury.

Sister Mary Frances is a Boston nun who had polio at two years of age. Her job in her convent is to tend to the aging nuns in her order and take them to their medical appointments. She came to see me because she was having pain in her legs and new weakness. When I initially evaluated Sister Mary, she reported that she occasionally fell; although this was often embarrassing to her (particularly when the priests had to help her up), she accepted such falls as part of her life. When I asked her to recount any injuries she had sustained during these "occasional" falls, the list was long and varied. Sister Mary reported among other things a fractured arm and wrist and multiple rib fractures. These had occurred separately, and on many other occasions she had sustained abrasions, lacerations, and bruises. Despite numerous injuries, Sister Mary had never worn a brace or used an assistive device. While she was being treated at our clinic, she began using a cane out in the community but declined to use one at home. She was also reluctant to consider any type of bracing. Sister Mary was a pleasure to treat; however, despite our rapport and the fact that I advised her to the contrary, she steadfastly clung to the idea that falling occasionally was unavoidable and therefore acceptable. Despite valiant efforts by the therapists and my own intervention, I am sure Sister Mary still believes this to be true.

MYTH 3. TRIPPING IS OKAY.

Many polio survivors have "foot drop," which may cause them to stumble and trip. *Tripping is less than a step away from a fall and is definitely not okay.* Even if a fall does not occur, the loss of balance incurred while tripping can result in an injury such as a sprained ankle. The polio survivor then has a new (albeit temporary) disability, which in turn makes further trips and falls more likely.

MYTH 4. IT IS NOT NECESSARY TO SEE A DOCTOR AFTER FALLING.

There are several reasons why an individual should consult his or her doctor after a fall. First, the possibility of a serious injury that may go undiagnosed without proper intervention is paramount. Some fractures of the bones are difficult to detect without an x-ray. Also, there may be bleeding internally, which cannot be detected without a formal physical examination and sometimes other studies such as a CT scan or an MRI. The classic example is a subdural hematoma, which is caused by bleeding of the small veins in the brain and can occur after someone hits his or her head. The person may feel fine initially, then begin to have signs of a problem more serious than originally suspected. These signs may include (but are not limited to) difficulty with balance, incontinence, difficulty with speech, and blurred vision.

Another reason to check in with the doctor after a fall is to evaluate what caused the fall. Sometimes a fall is the first sign of an underlying illness, which can be evaluated by a medical doctor. Often an undiagnosed infection is enough to cause someone to fall—especially if their strength and balance are not optimal under normal conditions.

MYTH 4. MOST FALLS OCCUR IN INCLEMENT WEATHER.

Many people believe that if they live in a warm climate and avoid going out in poor weather, they will not fall. As we have seen, most falls occur in a familiar environment and are not related to poor weather or risk-taking behaviors such as climbing a ladder.

MYTH 6. I WON'T FALL IF I STAY AT HOME.

As stated above, most falls occur at home, so staying in the house is not the solution. Further, this self-imposed isolation leads to depression and a reduced quality of life.

Preventing Falls

Preventing falls entirely is the only way to be certain to avoid serious injury (Table 16.3). To many polio survivors, the task may seem impossible; however, careful consideration of how to avoid falls will prevent most of them. Consider the following steps as a guide.

STEP 1. START WITH A CHECKUP BY YOUR DOCTOR.

Have your eyesight and hearing checked, as well as your blood pressure. Review your current medications and let the doctor know of any new medical problems.[10] Seek treatment for any painful

Table 16.3 Tips for preventing falls

Have a thorough medical checkup each year.
Discuss with your doctor any problems with medications, new injuries, and
   new symptoms such as fatigue, dizziness, or urinary frequency.
Have your eyes and ears checked regularly.
Have your braces and/or assistive devices checked and updated regularly.
Modify your home and workplace to make them safer.
Go out regularly, but avoid doing so when you are very tired or when the
   weather conditions are hazardous.
Exercise regularly, per your doctor's instructions, to improve flexibility,
   strength, balance, and coordination.

conditions that may cause you to be less steady than you usually are. Routine lab studies will reveal such factors as anemia, which may cause dizziness and subsequent loss of balance. Discuss treatment for osteoporosis and decide whether this is a viable option for you. Alert the doctor to any changes in your weight, because they may impact your mobility. Have your footwear and braces inspected during the visit as well; any problems with shoes, braces, or assistive devices should be evaluated and fixed.[11] Wheelchairs and scooters should be kept up to date and in good repair. Discuss your current exercise regimen. Keep in mind that people who exercise regularly can improve their balance and coordination, thereby helping to prevent falls.

STEP 2. LOOK AT YOUR HOME (AND WORK, IF
APPLICABLE) ENVIRONMENT.

Many insurance providers will cover the cost of a visit to your home or workplace by a physical or occupational therapist in order to address issues of safety and fall prevention. Even if your medical insurance does not cover this cost, it may be a wise investment. The

Table 16.4 Modifying your home and work environment to prevent falls

---

Repair cracked or broken stairs and walkways leading to building.

Have floor surfaces that are smooth but not slick. Get rid of raised thresholds and doorjambs. Get rid of throw rugs and clutter (e.g., exposed electrical cords, magazine racks).

Have sturdy stairs with handrails on both sides (indoors and outdoors). Consider getting a stair lift or elevator if going up and down stairs is difficult.

Sit only in sturdy chairs with armrests that are at a good height for you.

Sit on a sturdy chair or bench in the shower or bath. Have grab bars installed around the commode and in the bath/shower.

Use nonskid bathmats.

Maintain proper lighting throughout, but avoid glare.

Put all outlets and switches at arm's length to avoid reaching and bending.

Use a bedside commode or urinal at night.

Stabilize all furnishings, but avoid using the furniture to assist you in walking.

Store items at an accessible level to avoid reaching and bending.

---

advantages of having a therapist come to your home or workplace is that they will watch how you move about. Following a checklist such as the one provided in Table 16.4 is helpful, but cannot take the place of an expert who has the opportunity to evaluate you in your own environment.

With respect to your home, concentrate on being a minimalist and be sure your space is uncluttered. Avoid using furniture and other objects such as door handles and towel racks to support you. Be proactive and install protective equipment before you really need it (handrails for the stairs, grab bars for the bathroom). Have someone repair cracked or broken stairs and walkways. Get rid of raised thresholds, doorjambs, and scatter rugs. Consider installing a lift now rather than waiting until stair climbing becomes an unbearable burden.

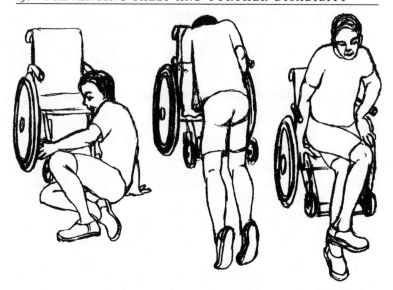

Figure 16.1 What to do after a fall. A. If your wheelchair is nearby, approach it in a forward position and use the front frame, seat, and/or back of the wheelchair to push yourself into it. Make sure the wheels are locked. Turn simultaneously to assume a balanced sitting position. B. If a bed or couch is handy, pull yourself onto the surface and lie on your stomach. When you have rested, roll onto your back or raise yourself to a seated position.

STEP 3. BALANCE THE PRECAUTIONARY MEASURES
TAKEN TO AVOID FALLING WITH MAINTENANCE
OF A GOOD QUALITY OF LIFE.

Instead of avoiding excursions, plan ahead so that you take rest breaks and avoid excessive fatigue. If a route is not easily accessible to you, consider asking for help rather than taking it on. Measure the price of independence with the risk of falling and choose the option that is best for you in a given situation. Keep in mind that a fall which causes a serious injury will invariably alter your independence and diminish your quality of life.

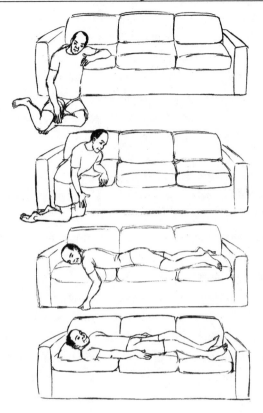

What to Do If You Do Fall

Not every fall can be prevented (although this should always be the goal), and it is worth taking time to consider what to do if a fall does occur. Ideally, someone will be nearby to assist you or call for help. Refer to Figure 16.1 for tips on how to get up after a fall and/or on how someone can assist you after a fall. Be prepared in the event that no one may be nearby to help. Wear either a medical alert device (commonly called a lifeline) or carry a portable phone in order to call for help.

If you have sustained any injuries as the result of your fall, you should contact your physician. Keep in mind that some injuries (such as a subdural hematoma or a bony fracture) cannot be seen without the special imaging studies ordered by a doctor. A good rule of thumb is to check with your doctor anytime you have fallen, particularly if you have hit your head. If you initially thought you had no injuries, but a few days later realize that you are sore and an area of your body is newly painful, contact your doctor and be evaluated. Treating injuries soon after they occur is much easier and more effective than treating them after several weeks or months have gone by. Maintaining the optimal level of function is imperative for your quality of life, and even minor soft-tissue injuries from a fall can dramatically change your ability to function. When in doubt, call your doctor.

Falls by polio survivors often lead to further disability. We have seen that most of them are preventable. Carefully considering your own history of slips, trips, and falls, then looking at both the intrinsic and extrinsic factors that contributed to these occurrences, will help prevent them in the future. Despite our best intentions, no one can guarantee that we will never fall. So have a plan in place in case you do fall. And keep in mind that early medical treatment is often the key to minimizing the injuries or disability incurred by a fall.

CHAPTER 17

Keeping Bones Healthy and Strong

Strong, healthy bones are essential to aging gracefully with polio and preserving the ability to function at the highest possible level. Unfortunately, when it comes to bones, paralytic polio survivors already have two strikes against them. The first is that bones surrounded by paralyzed muscles are generally not as thick and strong as bones surrounded by normally functioning muscles. A key element in maintaining the bones is the ability of strong muscles to contract and then relax (a perpetual tug and release process). The second strike is that polio survivors are not always able to perform the aggressive weight-bearing exercises that play a critical role in maintaining and sometimes improving bone density and strength. Aggressive weight-bearing exercises, even if polio survivors are physically able to perform them, may ultimately cause further weakness.

To avoid a third strike of any sort, it is absolutely imperative that polio survivors do everything they can to keep their bones in the best shape possible. Fortunately, there are many ways to help protect the bones and avoid the pain and disability that occurs with fractures. Keep in mind that the first step in treating any medical disorder is to recognize it as an issue that needs to be addressed.

Localized Osteoporosis

Localized osteoporosis may go unrecognized forever. On the other hand, a fracture may occur without warning or with minimal trauma.

Elizabeth (Betty) Smith is a seventy-year-old polio survivor who has led a physically active life. Her initial polio involved primarily her right arm, leaving her with some residual weakness there. One beautiful spring day, Betty and her husband decided to take a balloon trip with a guide and some other balloon enthusiasts. After a wonderful ride, the balloon landed with a thud and Betty was knocked into the woman standing next to her. Although she never fell, Betty hit her right arm against the other woman hard enough to break it. The other woman was shocked when Betty said that her arm was broken, since the force of the landing was nothing out of the ordinary. But because of Betty's history of polio and the localized bone loss in her right arm, she was highly susceptible to a fracture in this arm.

Polio survivors need to be aware that the bones in extremities that have some muscle paralysis are likely to be fragile and vulnerable to fracture.

Although polio survivors undoubtedly have some bone loss in paralyzed extremities (termed osteopenic or osteoporotic bones), they do not necessarily have *generalized* osteoporosis, which affects bones *throughout* the skeleton. In paralyzed limbs the bone loss applies only to where the paralysis occurred and for the purposes of this chapter will be termed *localized* osteoporosis. It is important to understand the distinction between *localized* and *generalized* osteoporosis. Anyone with paralysis almost certainly has bone loss in the region where the paralysis occurred; however, generalized osteoporosis has little to do with having had polio. The only risk factor for generalized osteoporosis that may be related to a history of having had polio is a sedentary lifestyle.

Polio survivors, particularly female polio survivors, certainly may have both generalized osteoporosis *and* localized bone loss. Generalized osteoporosis is the most common bone disease in the general population, and *all* polio survivors should do everything they can to prevent the further bone loss that occurs with generalized osteoporosis. Furthermore, regardless of whether someone has localized bone loss, generalized bone loss, or both, the end result (fragile bones vulnerable to fracture) is essentially the same.

There is not much someone can do about restoring localized bone loss that occurred decades ago due to paralysis from the initial polio; therefore, the remainder of this chapter will focus on two areas: (1) preventing fractures in polio survivors with localized bone loss, and (2) early diagnosis and treatment of generalized osteoporosis in polio survivors in order to prevent fractures and further disability. Most of the text will apply to polio survivors regardless of whether they have localized osteoporosis, generalized osteoporosis, or both. Occasionally some information will not apply to individuals who have localized bone loss exclusively, and this will be clearly stated so as to avoid confusion.

Generalized Osteoporosis

Osteoporosis has been called a silent disease, because it frequently progresses without symptoms. If the disease becomes severe, a fracture may occur with little or no trauma. Men and women of all races and nationalities are at risk for osteoporosis; however, *postmenopausal white women* have the highest incidence (13–18 percent are estimated to have osteoporosis, and 35 percent are estimated to have low bone density in the hip).[1] As you continue to read this chapter, keep in mind that most studies have focused on postmenopausal white women with *generalized* osteoporosis—therefore, the statistics have a built-in bias. Many of the studies have not taken into account persons with disabilities, persons of color, or men. This bias is well known and is currently being addressed by leading researchers.

One of the unfortunate results is that osteoporosis has been relegated to the status of a disease associated almost exclusively with women. Yet men too are at significant risk for osteoporosis.[2] One of the main consequences of the disease is a hip fracture, which can cause severe pain, disability, and even death; and men account for one-third of the total number of reported hip fractures.[3] Moreover, following a hip fracture men tend to have a higher incidence of disability and death than women do. *Therefore, early diagnosis of generalized osteoporosis is at least as critical for men as it is for women.*

Despite the notable deficiencies in the studies of osteoporosis, the statistics are impressive. In the *Physician's Guide to Prevention and Treatment of Osteoporosis,* published by the National Osteoporosis Foundation, osteoporosis is reported to be a disease that is reaching epidemic proportions in the elderly population: "Currently, an estimated ten million Americans suffer from osteoporosis and another eighteen million have low bone mass, putting them at risk for the pain and debilitation of fracture—one point five million each year, including 300,000 hip fractures, twenty percent of which lead to death within a year."[4]

The risk of fracture (with subsequent pain and disability) is much more likely in an individual with significant bone loss. The most common fractures occur in the hip, wrist or forearm, and spine (vertebrae). Fractures of the hip are usually the most serious and disabling. Consider that, in the general population, 15–20 percent of people who sustain a hip fracture will die within twelve months.[5] Moreover, 50 percent of people with a hip fracture will no longer be able to walk without assistance, and 20 percent will require long-term care (such as in a nursing home).[6] Although these statis-

Table 17.1 Tips on how to keep bones healthy

Eat a balanced diet rich in calcium and vitamin D.
Ask your doctor whether dietary supplements would be helpful.
Talk to your doctor about weight-bearing and muscle-strengthening exercises.
Avoid tobacco.
Limit alcohol.
Ask your doctor about bone-density testing and medication when appropriate.

tics are alarming, keep in mind that hip fractures are more common in the frail elderly, whose health is poor to begin with.

Fractures in the arms may be extremely disabling for polio survivors, who often rely heavily on their arms for mobility and for completing daily tasks independently. Fractures of the spine may be painful and lead to a stooped (kyphotic) posture. This type of posture may cause pressure on some of the body's internal organs, including the lungs. If this occurs, polio survivors may have difficulty breathing.

One of the questions I am asked frequently by polio survivors is, "Doctor, what is my long-term prognosis?" My answer is always that the symptoms of PPS tend to be very gradually progressive and with proper treatment may scarcely be noticeable. If a polio survivor sustains a fracture, however, the level of disability may change immediately and dramatically for the worse. Simply recognizing that bone injuries may lead to significant disability is the first step in protecting your bones. Table 17.1 gives some general guidelines on how to keep bones healthy.

PREVENTION OF GENERALIZED OSTEOPOROSIS

In order to prevent osteoporosis, we need to understand what causes the disease. Generalized osteoporosis, like Post-Polio Syndrome,

Table 17.2 Risk factors for bone fractures

Nonmodifiable:
History of paralytic polio
Having already had a fracture as an adult
Close family members (first-degree relatives) having had a fracture
Caucasian race
Advanced age
Female sex
Dementia
Poor health (frailty)

Potentially modifiable:
Currently smoking cigarettes
Underweight
Estrogen deficiency
Low calcium intake
Excessive alcohol consumption
Impaired eyesight (either not corrected or poor even with glasses, surgery, etc.)
History of falling
History of tripping
Inadequate physical activity
Poor health (frailty)

Note: Poor health (frailty) appears under both headings; it may or may not be modifiable.

does not have a single definable cause, but is the result of a variety of factors and influences—it is multifactiorial. The factors that often play a role include body weight, age, exercise history, diet, and an inherited predisposition to the disease. Obviously it is impossible to control the fact that some people are born with genes that make them susceptible to osteoporosis, but many of the other elements are *modifiable risk factors.* They are under our control and we are able to modify our lifestyle in order to make it less likely that we will get osteoporosis. Table 17.2 lists the common risk factors for fractures. In polio survivors, the most important modifiable risk factor is improving mobility and decreasing the risk of falls. Chapters 18–20 and 16 discuss these topics in detail.

Probably the risk factor most readily modifiable is the amount of calcium and vitamin D you are getting.[7] The National Osteoporosis Foundation recommends that you consume at least 1,200 milligrams each day of elemental calcium (including supplements if necessary) and 400–800 I.U. of vitamin D daily. Generally, the best way to get these nutrients is through diet. For instance, an 8-ounce glass of skim milk has 300 milligrams of calcium. Check to see if the milk you are drinking is also fortified with vitamin D, which helps calcium absorption. The same amount of yogurt, or 2 ounces of cheese, has 400 milligrams of calcium. Not everyone gets enough calcium and vitamin D in their diets, and even if a person does eat enough of these nutrients, other factors may affect how much the body is absorbing. Dietary supplements are often recommended. Check with you doctor to determine which supplements you may need.

A number of diseases are associated with generalized osteoporosis in both men and women. Early diagnosis and treatment in many instances will help to prevent bone loss. Table 17.3 lists diseases associated with an increased risk of generalized osteoporosis. The _long-term_ use of cigarettes, alcohol, and some medications may also increase the risk of generalized bone loss. Table 17.4 lists medications that may be associated with an increased risk of generalized osteoporosis. Most of the medications shown are used for serious and sometimes life-threatening medical conditions; therefore, despite the risk of bone loss, those medications may still be the best treatment for a particular condition. As always, discuss such concerns with your doctor.

DIAGNOSIS OF GENERALIZED OSTEOPOROSIS

It has long been known that low bone mass is one of the most reliable predictors of fracture. Therefore, in order to prevent fractures, it is important to identify individuals with low bone density.

Table 17.3 Diseases associated with an increased risk of generalized osteoporosis (National Osteoporosis Foundation list)

Acromegaly
Adrenal atrophy and Addison's disease
Amyloidosis
Ankylosing spondylitis
Chronic obstructive pulmonary disease
Congenital porphyria
Cushing's syndrome
Endometriosis
Epidermolysis bullosa
Gastrectomy
Gonadal insufficiency
Hemochromatosis
Hempohilia
Hyperparathyroidism
Hypophosphatasia
Idiopathic scoliosis
Insulin-dependent diabetes mellitus
Liver disease (severe)
Lymphoma
Leukemia
Malabsorption syndromes
Mastocytosis
Multiple myeloma
Multiple sclerosis
Nutritional disorders
Osteogenesis imperfecta
Parenteral nutrition
Pernicious anemia
Rheumatoid arthritis
Sarcoidosis
Thalassemia
Thyrotoxicosis
Tumor secretion of parathyroid hormone-related peptide

Table 17.4 Medications associated with an increased risk of generalized osteoporosis (National Osteoporosis Foundation list)

Aluminum
Anticonvulsants
Cytotoxic drugs
Glucocorticosteroids and adrenocorticotropin
Gonadotropin-releasing hormone agonists
Heparin
Lithium
Tamoxifen (premenopausal use)
Thyroxine (excessive)

The current guidelines regarding whom doctors should recommend for bone-density testing were not developed with polio survivors in mind. Thus, polio survivors should talk to their polio doctors about the risk of developing generalized osteoporosis and the advisability of having bone-density studies performed. I usually recommend to polio survivors that they have the testing done, and I refer them to rheumatologists or primary-care physicians who are skilled at ordering these tests and recommending appropriate treatment. Some polio doctors may prefer to do all the testing and treatment themselves. Who evaluates and treats a polio survivor for osteoporosis is irrelevant as long as that person has experience and informs any other physicians involved of the results of testing and any medication changes.

Fortunately, testing for osteoporosis is easy, painless, and affordable. The basic test is called a Bone Mineral Density (BMD) study. Its objective is to identify how dense bones are at different skeletal locations (hip, spine, and so on) in comparison to a "young normal" adult. The BMD measurements are statistically analyzed and an individual is labeled normal, osteopenic, or osteoporotic, depending on how much bone loss has occurred. The several different ways of measuring BMD are listed in Table 17.5.

Table 17.5 Bone mineral density tests

Dual-energy x-ray absorptiometry (DXA or DEXA)
    Can be done in a few minutes with radiation exposure that is
    approximately one-tenth that of a standard chest x-ray; measures bone
    density in the spine, hip, or wrist
Single-energy x-ray absorptiometry (SXA) and peripheral dual-energy x-ray
    absorptiometry (pDXA or pDEXA)
    Measures bone density in the forearm, finger, and heel
Radiographic absorptiometry (RA)
    Similar in accuracy and precision to SXA
Quantitative computed tomography (QCT)
    Most commonly used to measure bone in the spine
Ultrasound densitometry
    Measures bones that are superficial (e.g., heel and shin)

TREATMENT OF GENERALIZED OSTEOPOROSIS

The treatment of generalized osteoporosis varies depending on individual risk factors and medical conditions. However, some general recommendations apply to both men and women. Keep in mind that any treatable or curable medical condition that is causing bone loss should be addressed. Avoiding tobacco and limiting alcohol intake helps to prevent bone loss. Alcohol may also contribute to problems with balance and mobility, making falls more likely. Adequate intake of calcium and vitamin D is essential. Exercise may slow bone loss but will not restore bone that has already been lost. Exercise by polio survivors should always be done under the supervision of a polio doctor.

Medications may be used in both men and women to prevent and treat osteoporosis.[8] The traditional treatment has been hormone replacement therapy (HRT), which consists of testosterone in men and estrogen (often combined with progesterone) in women. Hormone replacement therapy is considered in men who have low testosterone levels and in women who are postmenopausal. In certain circumstances HRT is not advisable. For instance, it may not be recommended in men with a history of prostate cancer, or in either men or women with a history of breast cancer. Hormone replacement therapy may also not be appropriate for women who have a history of blood clots in their legs or who have a family member who has had breast cancer. Since HRT given to postmenopausal women may help to prevent heart disease, dementia, and some urologic diseases as well as osteoporosis, it should at least be *considered* in all postmenopausal women.

Hormone replacement therapy is not the only medication option for osteoporosis. Bisphosphonates are another class of medications that may be used in both preventing and treating osteoporosis. Calcitonin, a hormone produced by salmon that inhibits bone loss, is generally used as a nasal spray. Both calcitonin and bisphosphonates may be used in men and women, but their use has been more thoroughly studied in women. Both medications have been shown to *improve* bone density.

Also available for women is a class of compounds called selective estrogen receptor modulators (SERMS), which have many of the beneficial effects of estrogen without some of the disadvantages. This class of medications is generally used to *prevent* generalized osteoporosis, but in the future may be used more for *treating* the disease once it has developed. Remember that there is no perfect drug available to treat generalized osteoporosis, and anyone considering a medication regimen should consult with a doctor.

CHAPTER 18

Mobility

Mobility is one of the most meaningful topics for polio survivors to consider. Thus, the following three chapters are devoted to the subject. Three themes recur continually. The first is *safety*. Mobility should be safe, so that one does not risk falling and having a serious injury that may ultimately cause further disability. The second theme is *independence*. The goal should always be to encourage as much independence as possible—and mobility is a large part of independence. The third theme is *efficiency*—specifically, efficiency in the way one moves about. This is particularly important in polio survivors, who need to conserve energy and preserve strength.

In a perfect world, everyone could move safely, independently, and efficiently. Unfortunately, the world is not perfect and compromises must often be made in order to achieve mobility. For instance, a person may be able to walk independently (without using an assistive device such as a cane), but he may not be very safe and may risk falling. Even though the individual is reluctant to rely on an external device to assist him with mobility, he may need to compromise in order to be safe. Ultimately, each individual must decide what compromises he or she is willing to make in order to achieve the highest level of mobility.

The Spectrum of Mobility

Often when people think of being mobile, they think exclusively of walking; however, mobility involves much more than walking. Mobility issues include how an individual is able to position himself in bed, how he gets on and off the toilet, how he goes from his home to another location, and so on. In a polio clinic, mobility is a principal focus of treatment. When a rehabilitation specialist considers mobility issues in an individual, she wants to know the following: How is the individual moving from one place to another? How much assistance from another person does the individual need in order to move about? What equipment is currently being utilized to facilitate mobility? How safe is the individual when moving about? The goal of assessing a person's mobility status is to make all mobility as safe and easy as possible.

Although mobility involves much more than walking, a lot of the research done to date has centered on walking. We can extrapolate some of this information and apply it to transfers and wheelchair mobility as well. One of the key findings, repeated over and over, is that *any change or deviation from normal walking results in decreased efficiency and increased energy expenditure.*[1] Therefore, it is imperative to try and emulate "normal" mobility patterns insofar as possible. Another interesting finding is that individuals self-select their own most appropriate walking speed; somehow people know what pace is ideal for them. Changing that pace often results in the expenditure of additional energy. Studies have also shown that individuals are more efficient using assistive devices (crutches, canes, and the like) once they have practiced and become experienced with them. Other analyses have shown that carefully selecting an appropriate assistive device may markedly improve energy efficiency and safety.[2] For instance, it takes less energy to use a wheeled walker than a nonwheeled walker;[3] however, nonwheeled walkers are slower and safer to use. So if you need to use a walker for mobility, it is best to consult an expert on mobility issues so that the walker chosen will best suit your needs.

Another interesting though not surprising fact is that people who lose weight subsequently use less energy for mobility.[4] Less obvious is the fact that extra weight can actually affect the way in which a person walks. That is to say, significantly overweight individuals actually have altered foot and ankle motion, which leads to an abnormal gait pattern. Additionally, people who are overweight are more likely to develop arthritis of their joints, which also may affect how they walk if the knees and hips become painful.

As you can see, many factors impact a person's ability to move about. Therefore, improving mobility is a complicated task that requires careful analysis by knowledgeable experts. Polio survivors who have worked with experts generally report improvement in ease of walking, safety, and pain.

Recognizing Mobility Barriers

Many barriers affect an individual's ability to move safely and efficiently. Some are easily overcome, others may improve over time, and still others are permanent problems that need to be worked around. Barriers to mobility may be intrinsic to the individual, meaning that the mobility is hampered by a physical condition. On the other hand, barriers may be extrinsic to the individual, meaning that the environment adversely affects mobility. In polio survivors, the primary intrinsic barrier to safe and efficient mobility is weakness from the initial polio.[5] Frequently the initial weakness is worsened by symptoms of Post-Polio Syndrome. Although most polio survivors are not able to dramatically improve their strength, sometimes a subtle improvement in strength can make a big difference in *function.* For more on improving strength in polio survivors, review Chapter 13.

A common intrinsic mobility impediment occurs when muscles, tendons, and ligaments shorten—a process termed *contracture.* Contractures may occur in the extremities or the spine, and may significantly impede mobility or cause one to expend additional energy in order to compensate. Polio survivors frequently have contractures, which may improve with appropriately prescribed physical therapy. Contractures of the muscles and tendons of the hip and ankle are particularly problematic and often can be improved with physical therapy for a short period.

Other intrinsic mobility barriers include musculoskeletal pain, difficulty breathing, chest pain (angina), and dizziness (vertigo). It is important to seek medical attention from a physician if you are having pain or other symptoms that are affecting your mobility. Often the treatment is relatively simple and the results are gratifying.

Extrinsic factors that adversely affect mobility include floor surfaces that are slick, uneven, or have a high surface tension (such as thick carpets). Old, heavy, and worn braces and wheelchairs adversely affect mobility. Using an inappropriate assistive device such as an ill-fitting cane may have the same effect. Yet not using an assistive device at all may also hamper mobility. Poor weather conditions may make mobility more risky and less energy efficient. Lack of a stair rail or elevator may hinder mobility. An individual may have difficulty moving about in bed because of a mattress that is too soft or a bed that is too high. Getting on and off the toilet may be difficult when the seat is too low and grab bars are not available. There are many, many extrinsic factors that may hinder mobility. Fortunately, extrinsic barriers are often easy to improve or work around once they are recognized (see Table 18.1).

Table 18.1 Ten steps to improving safe, efficient, and independent mobility

---

1. Read all three mobility chapters in this book (Chapters 18–20), regardless of whether you currently need braces, a wheelchair or scooter, etc.
2. Protect your arms and keep them as healthy and as strong as possible.
3. Have your doctor evaluate and treat any painful conditions you have.
4. Consider using equipment that might improve your mobility and make you safer, more efficient, and more independent as well.
5. Update your current braces.
6. Don't use assistive devices (e.g., canes, crutches) unless they were specifically prescribed for you and are the correct device, size, etc.
7. Change your physical environment (your home and office if appropriate) in order to make mobility easier and safer. Remove or work around extrinsic mobility barriers. Consider having a home and/or office visit by a physical or occupational therapist who is an expert on the mobility issues of polio survivors.
8. Consider using a motorized wheelchair or scooter, particularly for long distances.
9. Obtain a formal mobility evaluation from a polio expert.
10. Follow through with the treatment recommended at your mobility evaluation (e.g., supervised physical therapy to improve contractures, using a different assistive device).

Your Arms and Your Mobility

Throughout this book I state repeatedly that one's arms are the keys to independence. The ability of individuals to use their arms is critical if they are to be able to bathe themselves, dress themselves, use the toilet, and so forth. Arm function is also vital to mobility, particularly in polio survivors who have had some paralysis of their legs. Arms are often the taken-for-granted workhorses that propel individuals from one place to the next. Consider for a moment the polio survivor who relies heavily on his crutches to move about. It is easy to see how much work is required of his arms as he uses them to advance the crutches and then swing his legs through. Think about what would happen if he had an injury to one of his arms that precluded use of the crutches. Most likely, he would cease to be ambulatory. Other forms of mobility would also be impacted. For instance, he would probably have difficulty getting up from the toilet with just one arm to use. He might have difficulty getting in and out of the car. A polio survivor with an injured arm may find himself unable to maintain his mobility alone despite having been independent essentially all of his life.

Although this example is rather dramatic, unfortunately it is the reality for some polio survivors. Other individuals may notice more subtle changes in their ability to move about when they have an injury to an arm. For instance, someone with a tendinitis may notice that she experiences more pain and more difficulty rising from a chair or the toilet. She may notice that it is difficult to go upstairs and hold onto the railing. Although her symptoms may be more subtle, they may lead to increasing difficulty with mobility and ultimately render her more disabled. As you consider mobility issues, keep in mind that for the majority of polio survivors the arms are critical. Also keep in mind that many upper-extremity injuries are treatable and sometimes even curable. For more information on preserving arm strength and function, see Chapter 6.

Mobility as a Form of Exercise

Encouraging people to use their mobility as a form of exercise has been recommended at one time or another by those of us in the health-care profession. For most people, it is a good idea: Take an extra flight of stairs. Walk or bike to work. Get off the bus two stops early and walk the rest of the way. Park your car at a distance and walk to the supermarket. And so on. For polio survivors, however, this advice should be treated with caution. The major problem with mobility as a form of exercise is that it is unpredictable. For instance, in a regimented exercise program one might use a stairclimber for a specific amount of time at a predetermined speed and incline. In contrast, an individual who is climbing stairs in an office building in order to exercise may go up and down five times one day and twenty times the next—depending, for instance, on where meetings are held. Similar examples apply to mobility in one's home and out in the community. For polio survivors at risk for further weakness from overuse, exercise ideally should be performed in a controlled manner.

Mobility issues are paramount in the lives of all of us as we age. Fortunately there are a number of actions that polio survivors can take to improve their mobility. And even if the next two chapters do not seem to apply to you just now, keep reading! All of us can benefit from stopping to consider how we are going to remain mobile and active as time goes on.

CHAPTER 19

Bracing, Shoes, and Assistive Devices

To many polio survivors the thought of using additional equipment (such as braces, wheelchairs, canes, or crutches), regardless of what they currently use, is unwelcome. Perhaps they view these devices as limiting their ability to do what they need to do rather than helping to make them more mobile and independent. Or some people may view the use of any type of equipment as an indication that they are disabled. They may be concerned about how others (particularly employers) will perceive such equipment. This perfectly rational concern sometimes results in vehement refusal to consider new or different bracing options, despite the fact that polio survivors may actually become more independent by using them.

People with the strongest adverse reactions may find that their feelings are historically based and date back to the time of their initial polio, when they were encouraged to use as little equipment as possible. During the polio epidemics of the first half of the twentieth century, people who became ill were instructed to "throw away" their braces and canes as soon as possible. The thinking then was that getting rid of any and all possible equipment meant recovery and was part of the road back to normalcy. Not getting rid of equipment was often equated with physical and moral failure. The less equipment individuals used, the greater their recovery and the more successful they were both personally and in their rehabilitation program. So deeply ingrained was the doctrine of discarding equipment that many survivors today view using any new device as "going back to being a cripple." Such thinking, which served numerous survivors well during their initial polio, is now causing some of the same individuals anxiety over what they should and should not be using to help with mobility.

The first section of this chapter discusses bracing. The terms *braces* and *orthotics* are used interchangeably to describe any type of device that is used to support and align an extremity. The second section focuses on shoes, and the third describes assistive devices. (The term *assistive devices* is used in this chapter to exclusively refer to mobility aids, which include canes, crutches, and walkers.)

Braces and Orthotics

The majority of paralytic polio survivors have worn some type of bracing since their illness. Many used the orthotics for only a short period (weeks to months) and then—thanks to recovery of paralyzed muscles, surgical procedures, or a combination of the two—they were able to walk without using braces. Other people were able to "downsize" from a long leg brace to a short one, or from two braces to one. Whatever an individual's experience, the common theme of "less is better and none is great" has been sounded to nearly everyone who has had polio. After all these years, why is the message changing? Or is it? In my polio clinic, the new message is this: Use as little equipment as possible, but do whatever is necessary to stay mobile and independent and *keep from falling!*

Let us go back for a moment to one of the examples in Chapter 16. John Melon had polio at four years of age, and after multiple surgeries was able to walk without braces or other assistive devices. At the time of John's initial evaluation with me, he had a sense that he was having more difficulty, but he could not articulate specific problems. Under further questioning, John revealed that he was falling several times each week and that his balance was quite poor. Initially opposed to any type of bracing, John eventually tried a very sleek, lightweight ankle-foot orthosis (also called an AFO or short leg brace). When in place, this brace was barely noticeable to a trained observer and virtually undetectable to the general public. Moreover, John became much more stable when he walked, and three years later reported that he had not fallen since he started wearing the brace. In this instance I prescribed the lightest and simplest orthotic that would keep John from falling. John also felt more comfortable and had more confidence when he walked. His limp was much less noticeable and he used less energy to walk.

Not every bracing story is an overwhelming success. However, as in the example above, bracing can make a significant difference both psychologically in terms of confidence and independence and physically by improving walking, standing, and transfers. In John's case, we were trying out a new brace that was lighter in weight than usual and was not made of the standard white plastic (polypropylene) from which many braces are fabricated. Initially the new material caused some problems; the brace actually broke in half shortly after John got it. Fortunately, the orthotist was able to fabricate a new brace that was nearly identical but much stronger and more durable. Obviously John, the orthotist, and I all wished that the initial brace had not broken, and we all worried that another incident might result in John's getting injured. Still, we recognized that bracing is often a process that involves trial and error—especially with something different from the more traditional heavy and bulky braces.

The five main types of bracing and orthotics options for polio survivors include (but are not strictly limited to) the following:

1. Simple shoe inserts or orthotics (which are not braces)
2. An ankle orthosis (AO), which is an ankle brace
3. An ankle-foot orthosis (AFO), which is generally known as a short leg brace
4. A knee orthosis (KO), which is a knee brace
5. A knee-ankle-foot orthosis (KAFO), which is generally known as a long leg brace.

All of these braces come either prefabricated or custom made. The main difference between a custom brace and a prefabricated brace is that the former is specifically made for a given individual and is generally more expensive than a similar brace that is made assembly style in large quantities to fit a number of people. A custom brace is not necessarily better; however, the likelihood is higher that it will achieve a close fit. This is particularly important for polio survivors, who often have foot and leg deformities due to paralysis, previous surgeries, and arthritis.

Not only do braces come prefabricated or custom made, but they are also made in many styles and from a variety of materials. Often people like to wear whatever they have worn in the past, even if it is bulky, heavy, and inefficient. I do not necessarily discourage this preference, primarily because getting used to a new type of brace is a long process to which a person must really be committed. However, I do always indicate what I think would be the lightest, most comfortable, safest, and most energy-efficient option. Then I encourage the person to decide whether to commit the time and energy required to learn to use something new.

Some of the materials used in bracing today are carbon composites that are lightweight and durable.[1] They may be employed for both short and long leg braces and both plastic and metal braces. Titanium (instead of aluminum or steel) may be used to make a brace lighter and more durable. These are just two examples of the modern materials that are being used. Unfortunately, they tend to be more expensive than the traditional materials and sometimes require additional effort by the patient and the orthotist in order to obtain a close fit. There is no perfect brace that works for everyone, but there are great braces that work for different individuals. The key to getting a suitable brace is finding an expert who is experienced in prescribing and making braces for polio survivors.

Regardless of the materials used in construction, and whether the brace is custom-made or prefabricated, each requires a formal prescription, ideally written by a doctor working closely with an orthotist. The outpatient center where I work has a specific time and day of the week when we have a bracing clinic for polio survivors. This clinic involves a physiatrist (polio doctor), an orthotist, and a physical therapist—who all give their opinions and collaborate on the type of bracing option that is best for a specific person. The individual who needs the brace is always present; we generally try a number of braces and observe the fit and how the individual moves with each one. Then we decide whether any of the prefabricated braces we have tried are sufficient, or whether customized bracing is desirable. If a customized brace is prescribed, the orthotist makes it in his shop. By the following week, the brace is ready and the individual tries it on in the clinic. Most adjustments can be made during the clinic; occasionally, more work is needed and the orthotist takes the device back to the shop. If a prefabricated brace is prescribed, minor adjustments are made during the initial fitting at the clinic, and the patient takes it home the same day. If more work needs to be done, the orthotist again takes the brace back to his shop and returns with it the following week.

This type of specialized clinic is the ideal way to be fitted for a new brace; however, it is undoubtedly not available to everyone. If not, a doctor can determine what type of brace is needed and write a prescription, which can then be taken to an orthotist at another location. If the doctor and the orthotist are experienced in treating polio survivors, the results should be fine. If either individual is inexperienced, however, the prescribed brace may not work well and it will sit unused in the closet. This scenario leaves the polio survivor without a brace, or in some instances with an old brace that may be too heavy or even broken. The skill and commitment required to fit someone properly is often underestimated; finding the best available resources is nearly always worth the effort.

The initial fitting is only the first step in prescribing an appropriate brace. The next step involves the individual's becoming accustomed to wearing the brace. I advise anyone with a new brace to start a "wearing schedule": he or she wears the brace briefly (less than one or two hours) for the first few days, then over the course of two to three weeks gradually increases the amount of time the brace is worn until it can be tolerated all day. If the brace is uncomfortable or causes any skin irritation, I advise the person to discontinue use immediately and come back to the bracing clinic.

Another step involves deciding whether an individual would benefit from formal gait training in physical therapy, and/or whether an assistive device such as a cane or walker is needed. These are clinical decisions that a polio doctor should make. I generally send individuals to physical therapy if they fit any one of the following criteria: (1) they have never worn a brace before, (2) the new brace is substantially different from their old brace, (3) on physical examination, they appear to need some additional gait training or help with transfers, (4) they have weakness or loss of range of motion that might be improved with physical therapy, or (5) they need to learn to use an assistive device properly.

Medical coverage for bracing varies with the individual insurance plan. In general, Medicare will cover 80 percent of any brace that is deemed medically necessary. Supplemental insurance will often pick up the final 20 percent of the cost. Other insurance plans run the gamut and cover anywhere from nothing to 100 percent of the cost of a brace. Frequently, written guidelines state that the insurance will cover one brace each year up to a specified amount of money. Regardless of who pays for the braces, they are generally fairly expensive and range from several hundred to several thousand dollars. Therefore, it is important to seek out experts who can prescribe an appropriate brace and fit the brace correctly the first time (generally with some modifications). If a brace does not fit well and cannot be used, the chances are that a new brace will have to be made at additional expense.

Shoe Options

Proper footwear is critical to improving one's mobility. Old, worn shoes are a hazard that may cause a person to use more energy while walking or even cause someone to trip and fall. Improper footwear, regardless of its age, may also cause pain in the feet, knees, hips, and low back. If worn for a prolonged period, it may cause or contribute to existing foot, ankle, and leg deformities. *Proper footwear, though often taken for granted, is an essential part of maintaining good health and preventing further disability.*

I am often asked, "Which shoes should I buy?" The answer is, "It depends." The truth is that there are no perfect shoes that will fit everyone well. As with bracing, finding suitable footwear is often a process of trial and error. The first consideration is where to find footwear. There are generally three options: (1) a community store that sells quality footwear in a variety of sizes and widths, (2) a store that specializes in shoes for persons with medical issues and employs on-site experts in fitting and modifying the shoes, or (3) a polio center that has a footwear clinic (often combined with the bracing clinic) and a shoe specialist on site.

For many people the first option is the simplest and most reasonable. It works best for those who do not require any modifications (lifts, inserts, and the like) to their shoes; they simply need shoes that are sturdy, lightweight, and fit well. People who need modifications may still choose the first option, then take the shoes to a shoe specialist. The other two options are probably simpler and ultimately may result in a better fit. Particularly for shoes that are connected to braces, it is advisable to get fitted where a shoe specialist is available on site. Both a cobbler and a pedorthist specialize in fitting and modifying shoes. Pedorthists work with individuals who have specific shoe needs owing to different medical conditions. Further, they have had formal training and have passed certification tests. Polio doctors should be able to give references to certified pedorthists.

Ideally, a person should consult a polio doctor for advice. A prescription is not always necessary, but it can be helpful in explaining to a shoe specialist what needs to be done. A prescription may also be useful for tax purposes. Sometimes shoes and/or modifications to shoes are covered by medical insurance, particularly if the shoes are attached to braces. Individuals with diabetes (who have specific shoe needs) may be eligible for reimbursement through their medical insurance (including Medicare).

Assistive Devices

Perhaps unfortunately, many assistive devices (canes, crutches, walkers) can be purchased at a local drug store. The convenience encourages people to purchase and use a device without knowing whether it is the right equipment for them, and without any formal fitting of the device and training in how to use it. Consider the following questions on the use of a cane: In which hand should a cane be held—on the same side or opposite to the affected leg? If both legs are affected, should one use two canes, or switch to a walker or crutches? Which leg is advanced simultaneously with the cane? How long should the cane be? Should it be a single-point cane or a four-point (quad) cane?

As you can see, even the simplest assistive device (a cane) generates a number of questions. This is why it is critical to have any assistive device formally prescribed by an expert. Moreover, physical therapy may be necessary in order to teach proper use of the device. The downside of using a cane improperly is significant and involves the following potential problems: increased energy expenditure for mobility, increased pain and potential injury to the legs and back, increased risk of falling, and development of poor gait patterns that are difficult to unlearn—even with physical therapy at a later date!

To reiterate, *all assistive devices should be prescribed by a medical doctor or physical therapist who is an expert in treating polio survivors and who understands their gait mechanics, transfers, and other mobility issues.* A formal fitting should take place, and sometimes formal gait training in physical therapy is beneficial.

Acquiring properly prescribed and fitted braces, shoes, and assistive devices requires time, effort, and the advice of polio experts. Although there is often a period of trial and error and sometimes people's needs change over time, properly prescribed mobility devices can improve transfers, standing, and walking. They can improve balance and decrease pain and energy consumption. They can lessen the risk of falling. Furthermore, improving mobility has positive psychological benefits, including an increase in confidence, independence, and quality of life.

CHAPTER 20

Wheelchairs and Scooters

Many polio survivors have used a wheelchair or a motorized scooter since the time of their initial polio. Others are finding that due to weakness and decreased endurance from Post-Polio Syndrome they need help for long-distance mobility (particularly out in the community). Although few people who have never utilized a wheelchair or scooter relish the idea of using one, these appliances can significantly improve their quality of life and open a whole new world to individuals whose environment is becoming limited because of mobility issues. Countless polio survivors have told me that they no longer go to places they enjoy because they are unable to walk there safely and comfortably. Sometimes they do not visit family members, including children and grandchildren; travel for business or pleasure may be curtailed; even going to the mall may become too cumbersome. A wheelchair or scooter may be a lifesaver for polio survivors whose mobility is not what it used to be.

Regina Woods is a polio survivor who had significant residual paralysis following her acute polio. She describes her first experience with a motorized wheelchair: "For the first time since the onset of polio, I could move to a different area of my room without a word to anyone. I could move closer to my mother in order to hear her better. I could go into another room to hassle Gerry [her sister]. I was soon learning that there was a whole new world right there inside my house, as I saw things I had never before even noticed."[1]

Regina is at one end of the spectrum in that she had marked paralysis that remained after her initial polio, and a motorized wheelchair afforded her the opportunity to quite literally see a world that she had not seen for decades. But wheelchairs and scooters are not only for polio survivors who have severe paralysis and cannot walk. They may be useful for many polio survivors—depending on mobility needs, endurance, level of weakness, and so on. Yet many polio survivors fear that if they use a wheelchair or scooter for mobility, even part-time, they will become so dependent on the device that they will lose their ability to walk altogether. In fact, just the opposite is true. Polio survivors who can walk but are experiencing difficulty, particularly with long distances, actually have a better chance of preserving their ability to walk if they limit the overuse of their muscles by employing a wheelchair or scooter. For example, polio expert and survivor Lauro Halstead walks quite well, but for years has used a motorized scooter at work in order to avoid stressing the muscles in his legs by walking the long hospital corridors. Dr. Halstead uses the scooter for long distances in order to save his strength and energy, then parks it and walks in and out of patients' rooms, nursing stations, and the hospital cafeteria.

Although both Regina Woods and Lauro Halstead own their vehicles, sometimes polio survivors do not need to have one at their disposal at all times.

Ann Woods was a woman in her midforties whom I had the oppor-
tunity to see when I was in Washington, D.C., training under Dr.
Halstead. Ann came to the polio clinic because she was having difficulty
walking long distances and it was affecting her hectic life as a govern-
ment executive. One of Ann's primary concerns was that she had to

curtail her air travel, since she could not manage the long corridors she had to walk in the airports. She had never used any braces or mobility devices following her initial polio. Although she was having trouble walking and was experiencing some falls, Ann was taken aback when the team at the clinic suggested she consider wearing a short leg brace and using a scooter. Ann initially went home discouraged, but after several days she realized that she needed to make some concessions if she wanted to keep the job she loved. When she came back to the clinic, she agreed to try a brace (that she eventually became quite fond of) and to use a borrowed scooter at malls, airports, amusement parks, and other places where she needed to go farther than her legs could reasonably take her. The goal was to help Ann decrease the amount of stress she was placing on her leg muscles and to keep her from falling and incurring an injury.

The Manual versus Motorized Debate

I am often asked whether it is better to get a manual wheelchair (one that you propel with your arms) or a motorized one. My standard answer to this dilemma is, *Always get a motorized wheelchair or scooter unless someone else is going to push you in a manual chair.* Not everyone would agree with this statement; however, I staunchly defend it. The key to anyone's independence is their ability to use their arms. Consider two people with spinal cord injuries—one who is injured in the lumbar (low-back) area and has lost the use of his legs but his arms are completely spared, and the other who has a central cord injury in which his arms are paralyzed but his legs are strong. Which of these two people will be independent? The answer is the person whose arms are spared, because *you need your arms to be independent.*

What does this have to do with polio survivors? After all, if a polio survivor has strong arms, then using a manual wheelchair seems to make sense. The problem is twofold: (1) he or she risks overuse of the arms in a manual-style wheelchair, which can lead to permanent weakness, and (2) he or she risks injuring the arms (shoulder injuries and nerve injuries are more common in polio survivors than in the general population owing to the stress on their arms during daily activities) and thus fundamentally risks the ability to be independent. In my opinion, protecting a polio survivor's arms is crucial and using a manual wheelchair to propel oneself is a hazard. Keep in mind that most polio survivors who have paralysis in their legs do not have normal reserves of strength in their arms. The polio virus generally attacks more than 95 percent of the anterior horn cells in the spinal cord, and while the arms may be significantly stronger than the legs, they almost always are affected to some degree and therefore need additional protection.

A second reason why I favor motorized vehicles is that they allow polio survivors to go farther and thereby make it more convenient to go where they want to go and do what they want to do. The major drawback is that motorized mobility devices are heavier than manual chairs and need special equipment to transport them. Someone can fold up a manual chair and put it into the trunk or backseat of a car, whereas a motorized scooter or wheelchair needs a special lift. Transport of these devices today is getting much easier, as the newer lifts are more durable and convenient. Vans, often used to transport wheelchairs and scooters, are also more widely available.

One of the comments I commonly hear is that people want to use a manual chair in order to keep their upper body strong and in good condition. In theory this is a fine idea, but in practice using a wheelchair as a form of exercise is not very practical and may lead to some of the problems described above. I urge polio survivors instead to develop an appropriate upper-body conditioning program that they perform regularly. Each muscle group thereby can be worked appropriately without overusing one and underusing another (a phenomenon that occurs when someone performs the same repetitive motions such as propelling a wheelchair). Also, an appropriate exercise program is designed to be self-limiting in both intensity and duration, whereas propelling a manual wheelchair depends on where individuals need to go on a particular day. They may get a lot of exercise (if they have many places to go) or not much exercise at all. My point is that any form of exercise should be regulated in polio survivors, not left to chance.

Selection of a Wheelchair or Scooter

The process of getting a new wheelchair or scooter can be daunting, if not discouraging. There are ways to make the ordeal go more smoothly, however. I recommend that anyone purchasing a new motorized mobility device go to a mobility seating clinic if at all possible. These clinics are generally found at major rehabilitation hospitals and medical centers. It is definitely worth the time and effort to try to find one in your area. Prior to developing a wheelchair and scooter seating clinic as part of our polio clinic, I found that people were getting quite a variety of motorized vehicles. Some were excellent pieces of equipment, but not right for the person or they fit poorly. Sometimes the vendor had talked the individual into a lot of unnecessary extras or sometimes had not given the person the extras needed. Even with a written prescription (usually a requirement in order to have part or all of the cost covered by a medical insurer), problems arose. I realized that the problems were not being sufficiently addressed by the vendors because they were accountable to no one. In a clinic, if the vendor wants to continue to work there (which certainly can be lucrative), then that person needs to take care of all the problems that arise with past or present devices.

The wheelchair and scooter seating clinic where I work starts with an initial evaluation by the physical therapist and the polio doctor. The physical therapist then contacts the vendor and sets up a time when he or she can bring models of the types of motorized devices that are likely to suit the patient's needs. The people involved in the clinic include the polio survivor, the vendor, the physical therapist, and the doctor. During the clinic the patient has the opportunity to sit in different wheelchairs and/or scooters and try them out. She or he can look at different modifications or special features before ordering them. At the end of the clinic, the physical therapist writes out a detailed prescription for the desired wheelchair or scooter, with all the modifications and specialized features required. The physician then signs the prescription.

Prior to scheduling an appointment in the seating clinic, the physical therapist frequently makes a home visit. Such a visit can be infinitely helpful in determining how useful a wheelchair might be in the home, and which modifications might make it easier to use (for instance, installing a ramp to the front door, widening the bathroom doorway, rearranging furniture, or checking the height of the bed and toilet for transfers).

Although a seating clinic is the ideal way to be fitted for a wheelchair or scooter, there are other options. These include meeting with your polio doctor or a physical therapist who is knowledgeable about how to order mobility devices, and looking through catalogs. If you find what you want in a catalog, often you can arrange with the vendor to have a trial in your home or in his shop. In most instances, for insurance purposes you will need a written prescription from a physician that includes a justification based on your medical history and diagnosis, as well as a detailed description of the recommended appliance. Thus, at some point your polio doctor will need to be involved in the process.

WHEELCHAIR COMPONENTS

Getting fitted for a wheelchair involves a number of considerations. These include, but are not limited to:

1. Will the wheelchair be used indoors and outdoors?
2. Is extra space needed for braces (orthotics)?
3. Is a heavy-duty frame required (generally for a person heavier than 250 pounds)?
4. What types of table surfaces will be needed for home and office (are desk arms necessary)?
5. What accommodations are needed to obtain optimal seating posture?
6. Is a pressure cushion necessary?
7. How will transfers be accomplished?
8. How will the wheelchair be transported to a different location?

These are general questions that need to be considered by someone experienced in prescribing wheelchairs; however, a basic understanding of wheelchair components is useful.

Externally powered wheelchairs (motorized) consist of a drive system, a battery power source, and an operator controller system. When considering what type of motorized wheelchair to get, you should first determine whether the chair will be primarily used indoors or outdoors. Indoor chairs are slower, lighter, and easier to maneuver. They are generally less expensive than outdoor chairs, which are heavier, bulkier, and faster. Using an indoor chair outdoors will shorten its life expectancy, while using an outdoor chair indoors can be awkward. Many people want a combination chair that will work indoors and outdoors, and although there is no perfect chair, some can provide a nice compromise. The controller system for a motorized wheelchair can be operated with a joystick, a chin control, or even a puff-and-sip system (for quadriplegics who use breathing techniques to control the chair's movements). Although these systems may be sold separately, it is best to try and get everything from the same vendor, in order to limit the complications that can arise when a chair needs to be fixed or a new part ordered.

The basic component of any wheelchair is the frame. There are many to choose from, and the type that best suits someone will depend on the user's height and weight, sitting posture, transfer technique, and ability to use different types of controls to operate the chair.

Attached to the frame is a variety of options. The first is a seat belt, used for safety and for aligning the pelvis and improving sitting posture. As with all components, there are many different versions to choose from. The next attachments to the base are those that position and support the legs and feet. Many polio survivors need specialized front riggings and foot plates in order to accommodate leg, ankle, and foot deformities. Rear tires and wheels are two separate components and incorporate features such as weight and durability. The tires surround the wheels and consist of three general types—solid, pneumatic (air filled), and airless (solid insert). If pneumatic tires are ordered, an air pump can be added to the prescription. Handrims are mounted on the rear wheels and are used for self-propulsion in a manual chair. Casters are the small front wheels that allow the chair to turn and change directions. The tires for the casters can be pneumatic, semipneumatic, or solid (rubber). Wheel locks can be toggle or lever style.

Individuals frequently experience problems with armrests, which are important because among other things they impact transfers, the ability to sit close to a specific table surface, and the width of a wheelchair. Occasionally armrests are not necessary at all. For transfers, one might find swing-away or removable armrests easier to use. Desk arms are shorter and allow one to sit comfortably at a desk or table. The height of the armrests is a significant comfort and safety issue. The padding can affect how much pressure is placed on sensitive areas in the upper extremities that may be vulnerable to nerve injuries (such as an ulnar neuropathy at the elbow). The armrests also contribute to the ultimate width of the chair, which can affect ease of maneuvering doorways and overall turning radius. A lap board may be useful to rest the arms and to provide a table surface in order to write, eat, or read.

Sitting posture varies with an individual's strength and the presence of any structural deformities (such as scoliosis). Seat inserts can provide postural support for the pelvis, hips, and legs. Back, neck, and trunk supports provide postural support for the spine and trunk. Seat cushions provide comfort and reduce pressure from prolonged sitting. They can be ordered with a protective covering if incontinence is an issue; it may be advisable to order two seat covers so that a spare is available when one is laundered.

Storage containers such as a wheelchair pack can also be ordered to fit a particular chair. Sometimes baskets are used for storage. The initial evaluation (prior to obtaining the written prescription) is the time to consider all of these wheelchair components, including storage compartments.

SCOOTER COMPONENTS

Motorized scooters or carts have several advantages over motorized wheelchairs in terms of aesthetics and style, long-distance range, and suspension and power equipped to handle rough terrain. Use of a scooter requires reasonably good posture and upper-body strength. Thus, for someone with poor posture and upper-body strength, a motorized wheelchair will give more support and is a better choice.

Front-wheel-drive scooters are smaller than rear-wheel-drive scooters and therefore are more maneuverable and able to turn in smaller spaces. However, rear-wheel-drive scooters have better traction and will drive more easily through uneven surfaces and up and down hills. All front-wheel-drive systems use either a belt and chain or two belts to turn the front wheel. Rear-wheel scooters have multiple systems including the direct-gear drive, which is the smoothest, quietest, and most durable.

Scooter frames come in a variety of styles. Modular frames can be broken down into several different parts for ease of transport. One-piece frames will fit into most car trunks but require an electric lift (or someone to heft 100–150 pounds into the trunk). Scooter seats provide different levels of comfort and support. A unique feature of scooters is that their seats come with a 360-degree swivel, to facilitate getting on and off. When trying out a scooter, check the seat and determine whether you can easily engage and disengage the lock. Armrests are optional, but can provide additional stability and postural support. All scooters come with a battery charger, which can be of various types. As with wheelchairs, storage accessories can be purchased at the time the scooter is ordered. Once again, it is best to discuss the different scooter components with a physical therapist, a polio doctor, and a vendor prior to purchase.

COMMON WHEELCHAIR AND SCOOTER PROBLEMS

The following list addresses common wheelchair and scooter problems that are generally easily fixed.

1. The vehicle is uncomfortable. This is generally caused by a poor original fit (the seat back is too low, the seat is too high, the footrests are too low and scrape the ground going up curbs, and so on).

2. It is easy to slide out of the seat. Some of the reasons include poor initial fit, seat belt is broken or too loose, seat is too short or long, footrests are too low and do not support feet, and hamstrings are tight.

3. The body leans to one side or is slumped in the seat. This problem often results from weakness and postural problems, and can frequently be corrected with additional supports.

4. The wheelchair is too small or too big, often a difficulty when someone has a very old wheelchair, has lost or gained a lot of weight, or is using someone else's vehicle.

5. The brakes do not work or are hard to set. The parts may be worn, or a brake extension may be required.

6. The appliance is not moving well. The problem may be flat tires, a worn battery, or terrain that is too difficult for the chair.

7. It is difficult to have the appliance fixed. During the life of the scooter or wheelchair, repairs will inevitably need to be made. Once again, going to a formal seating clinic helps to ensure that the vendor will be responsive. (Some vendors will allow individuals to borrow another appliance until theirs is fixed.)

8. Armrests get in the way or do not assist with transfers. The initial appliance fitting should take into consideration how someone is going to transfer. The armrests often play a critical role in helping or hindering that ability.

FOUR STEPS TO PURCHASING AND REPAIRING A
POWER-OPERATED VEHICLE

1. Set up an appointment at a seating clinic, with your doctor, or with a participating vendor. As discussed above, fewer problems are likely if you can find a seating clinic. The advantages include: (a) knowledgeable physicians and therapists who will fit you properly for a vehicle without any financial incentive (a vendor is often paid on commission, whereas the medical experts at a seating clinic are paid a flat fee that is covered in the same manner as an office visit), (b) people who can help with the insurance paperwork, and sometimes will even file it for you, and (c) repairs and modifications

are easier when you go back to the seating clinic where you initially got the appliance.

2. Once you have decided on a vehicle, obtain a written quote from the vendor. Ideally, the vendor should be able to tell you how much your insurance will cover and how much you will ultimately be responsible for. You should call your medical insurer to verify the coverage, because the amount insurance plans will cover on a power-operated vehicle varies from zero to 100 percent.

3. The paperwork you need to obtain will vary depending on your medical insurance. For Medicare you will need the following: (a) a certificate of medical necessity (CMN), which must be filled out by a specialist in physical medicine and rehabilitation, orthopedic surgery, neurology, or rheumatology. If you are not able to have one of these specialists fill out the form for you, additional documentation must accompany the CMN to show why this is the case (you do not need a CMN if you have a prior approval number); (b) an insurance claim form, HCFA 1500 (you need to fill out items 1–14, your doctor fills out items 17, 17A, and 21, and the vendor fills out the rest; (c) a notepad prescription from your doctor; (d) a copy of your Medicare card; and (e) a copy of your receipt to be submitted for reimbursement.

4. Repairs to power-operated vehicles are frequently covered by medical insurance if it paid for the initial vehicle; you must have a prescription stating what is required and that it is medically necessary for your particular condition.

In summary, motorized wheelchairs and scooters may significantly improve polio survivors' quality of life, even if they are only used occasionally. The goal is always to give a person more freedom to move about, thereby increasing his or her independence. If you are interested in exploring these mobility options, try them out at the local grocery store or mall, then talk to your polio doctor about your needs and desires.

CHAPTER 21

Surgical Considerations

Surgery can be an ominous and intimidating prospect for someone who has had polio. Childhood memories of surgical procedures that were painful and frightening may still haunt polio survivors who are now adults. On the other hand, many polio survivors experienced great success with surgery after the acute polio. For instance, a successful muscle transplant that allowed someone to walk without braces may be fondly recalled. Surgery may be a welcome thought to many polio survivors as they envision vast improvements in their current health status. Regardless of whether one contemplates surgery with enthusiasm or trepidation, being aware of the risks and benefits of any surgical procedure is essential.

When the prospect of surgery is being contemplated, four main stages in the process need to be addressed: *preoperative planning, operative concerns, immediate postoperative recovery, and rehabilitation.*

Preoperative Planning

Apart from the skill of the surgeon's hands in the operating room, careful preoperative planning is the key to a successful surgery. Five steps are involved in that planning.

STEP 1. DECIDE WHETHER THE SURGERY IS NECESSARY.

This may seem obvious; however, many surgeries are *elective* and may not be absolutely necessary. If a life-threatening situation occurs that requires surgical intervention, then the focus shifts quickly to preparing for the surgery. If, however, the surgery is not being performed to meet a crisis condition, then several other things should be weighed. First, consider whether the medical condition can be treated by other means (for example, can medications be prescribed to control the symptoms?). Second, ask the surgeon what the chances are that the surgery will be successful. Third, decide whether a second opinion might be helpful.

Eileen O'Malley is a sixty-five-year-old woman who had polio when she was twelve. She initially recovered the strength in her legs quite well and never used any braces or assistive devices. Recently, however, Eileen began falling and noticed that her right knee was becoming increasingly painful—possibly contributing to her falls. An orthopedist told Eileen that she has severe arthritis and needs to have the knee replaced. As an alternative, Eileen came to the polio clinic to see if she could avoid surgery. Because she had not yet tried any treatment for her knee, she was given oral anti-inflammatory medications and referred to physical therapy, where she underwent some gentle strengthening exercises of the muscles surrounding the knee. The physical therapist fitted her with a knee brace and showed her how to "unload" the right knee by walking with a cane. Within a few weeks, Eileen was walking without significant pain and was no longer falling. She felt more confident and stable with the cane and knee brace and decided not to pursue the knee replacement.

Eileen had multiple options for nonsurgical treatment. Even though her surgery would have been elective, she might have gone through with the knee replacement if the interventions offered her at the polio clinic had not worked. Remember that it is important to consider the *nonsurgical* options as well as the *surgical* options.

STEP 2. TALK TO THE SURGEON AND THE SURGICAL TEAM.

Economic constraints have greatly changed surgical preoperative and postoperative routines. Same-day surgeries (in which the patient is admitted to the hospital and discharged on the same day) and outpatient surgeries are increasingly common, and the first opportunity a patient has to meet the surgical team may literally be minutes before being rolled into the operating room! Thus, someone with a history of polio who is scheduled for surgery will need to make a special effort to contact members of the surgical team prior to the operation.

The surgical team generally consists of operating-room and recovery-room nurses and at least one surgeon and anesthesiologist or nurse anesthetist (who works under the supervision of the anesthesiologist). Most issues surrounding the surgery should be discussed with the surgeon prior to arriving at the hospital; however, arriving early to talk to the anesthesiologist and/or nurses on duty is advisable.

Ask the surgeon well in advance how extensive the surgery will be, and what type of setting would be best. Can the operation be performed under local anesthesia in the surgeon's office (outpatient surgery)? If not, can it be done with a regional anesthetic block (numbing just one arm or leg), or as a same-day surgery with a spinal or epidural block? Can the surgery be done less invasively, using a laparoscope instead of making a larger incision? Advances in technology such as laser or laporoscopic surgery have in many instances made surgical procedures much simpler, with a shorter recovery time and fewer complications. Obviously, the primary concern when undergoing surgery is to achieve the surgical goals and limit the complications as much as possible. While the issues listed above are important to raise, ultimately the surgeon's experience and level of comfort with any given procedure is critical to the success of the surgery. Addressing these issues is a useful way to open up dialogue with the surgeon, but should not be used to override the surgeon's instincts or skill in a particular area.

The surgeon should be aware that the respiratory muscles of many persons with a history of polio have been involved (even if the individuals have never experienced any breathing problems and never used an iron lung). Thus, a simple preoperative study that should routinely be ordered for any polio survivor undergoing general anesthesia is *pulmonary function tests* (PFTs). These studies can be useful to determine baseline lung function, and may be helpful in anticipating any respiratory complications of the surgery.

Individuals with significant paralysis may have less blood volume than expected and may need a transfusion. Deciding whether to bank one's own blood or consider using donor-directed blood should be discussed with the surgeon prior to scheduling the surgery.

The anesthesiologist or nurse anesthetist is responsible for the type and the amount of anesthesia that will be administered. Part of the anesthesiologist's job is to talk to the patient before going to the operating room about the risks of anesthesia, and then to obtain a signed consent for the type of anesthesia selected. This is the time to address any concerns about anesthesia. Although the scientific literature regarding anesthesia and persons with a history of polio is sparse, many experts believe that anesthesia, particularly general anesthesia, may have a pronounced, perhaps deleterious effect. The reasons are ambiguous but may have to do with the nerves having been affected by the initial polio. As a general rule, persons who have had polio require lower doses of anesthesia and need longer before the anesthesia wears off. Reviewing this prospect with the anesthesiologist prior to surgery may be valuable.

If general anesthesia is to be used, the anesthesiologist should review the pulmonary function tests prior to surgery as well.

STEP 3. PLAN FOR DISCHARGE AFTER THE SURGERY.

Planning for discharge before the surgery even occurs may seem a bit premature; however, a little forethought can ease the transition. Depending on the hospital's policies and staffing, discharge planning may be the responsibility of the surgeon, the floor nurse, or the social worker.

Now is when decisions regarding rehabilitation should be made. Taking the time to talk to whoever is responsible for coordinating the discharge to one's home or to another facility for rehabilitation is ideally done before surgery.

STEP 4. ARRANGE PERSONAL AND BUSINESS AFFAIRS.

Few people will enter a hospital to undergo surgery without feelings of anxiety and trepidation. In order to focus on the surgery without worrying about what is *not* being done at home, arrange for someone to pay the bills, care for the dog, collect the mail, and attend to other chores.

STEP 5. CHOOSE A REHABILITATION PLAN.

If rehabilitation is expected to be necessary following a surgery, it is best to choose the most appropriate and useful type of treatment before the surgery takes place. (Rehabilitation options are described later in this chapter.) Deciding on which rehabilitation option is most beneficial will allow for a faster recovery. And planning ahead will help to ensure that one's health insurance is adequate to cover the anticipated medical expenses. Ideally in a surgery where rehabilitation is expected to be a major part of the recovery, the patient will meet with the therapists *preoperatively* to go over treatment plans and equipment needs.

Thomas Brown is a polio survivor who fell on an icy driveway during the winter. Unfortunately, he broke the right hip on his "polio side" (the right leg was most affected by the polio) and was taken by ambulance to a local hospital where he underwent surgery almost immediately to stabilize the fracture. Six months later, Tom began complaining of severe pain in his left hip. After a consultation at the polio clinic, he was referred to an orthopedist for consideration of a left total hip replacement. Although Tom had occasionally complained of left hip pain in the past, when he broke his right hip he became even more dependent on his "good leg." The arthritis in the left hip that had developed over the years significantly worsened after his fall. Tom decided to have the surgery, but first made arrangements for his postoperative rehabilitation. After deciding where he would go for this treatment, he met with the physical and occupational therapists. The physical therapist told Tom to expect that he would need to use a walker to ambulate for the first few weeks, then he would progress to a cane. She fitted him with a walker and showed him how to use it. The occupational therapist gave Tom a list of equipment he would need to purchase for his home, including a raised toilet seat and grab bars for his bathroom. Grateful for the recommendations, Tom left feeling reassured and ready for his upcoming surgery. Tom had the hip replacement and completed his rehabilitation within ten weeks.

Operative Concerns

We have seen that many aspects of a surgery should be discussed well before entering the operating room—anesthesia, possible blood transfusions, and the like. Other operative concerns include positioning of the patient during the surgery. Some people with a history of polio have had spinal surgeries and may have rods in their backs. Improper placement of those individuals during surgery can result in severe back pain.

Even if someone has not had spinal surgery, paralysis may cause the bones to have become brittle; proper positioning on the operating table can be critical. Because patients are generally positioned by the surgical team after being anesthetized (and are therefore unconscious), persons with a history of polio may want to request that they be positioned while still awake, in order to avoid uncomfortable and/or potentially harmful positions.

Immediate Postoperative Recovery

Once again, many of the issues that affect the immediate postoperative period should be discussed during the preoperative planning stages. These include ensuring that the recovery-room nurses are aware that persons with a history of polio may be slow to come out of anesthesia. Because polio survivors may be more sensitive to pain than others, they may require more than the usual amount of narcotic medication after surgery. Many postoperative orders are listed on a standard form and are simply checked off by the surgeon without necessarily considering the individual needs of the patient; therefore, discussing postoperative pain control prior to surgery is beneficial.

Furthermore, polio survivors may be particularly sensitive to cold owing to an inability to effectively regulate their body temperature. Many have complained of severe discomfort after waking up in the recovery room bitterly cold and shaking violently. Requesting extra blankets (or blankets that are prewarmed) in advance can help to avoid this uncomfortable experience.

Rehabilitation

For all but very minor procedures, most persons with a history of polio who are undergoing surgery will need some type of rehabilitation. There are four basic types: acute rehabilitation hospitalization, subacute rehabilitation hospitalization, rehabilitation at home, and outpatient rehabilitation.

ACUTE REHABILITATION HOSPITALIZATION

This is the most aggressive and comprehensive type of rehabilitation. Once individuals are discharged from the hospital where they had surgery, they immediately go to another hospital (or sometimes to another part of the same hospital), where they participate in an intensive rehabilitation program. The highly trained rehabilitation teams include doctors (generally physiatrists and other medical consultants), rehabilitation nurses, physical and occupational therapists, speech and language pathologists, orthotists (brace makers) and prosthetists (artificial-limb makers), social workers, psychologists, vocational counselors, and recreational therapists. Although most patients will not need all of these services, the availability of a wide array of rehabilitation professionals is a distinct advantage.

While this arrangement may sound ideal, certain factors may eliminate an acute rehabilitation hospitalization as an option. For example, medical insurance guidelines often limit who can go to these types of settings. Generally, an appropriate patient is someone who has had a complicated surgery with an expected long recovery period and needs intensive therapy on a daily basis. The guidelines usually state that the patient must be able to tolerate at least three hours a day of physical and occupational therapy. Even though this regimen is split up over the course of the day, many people cannot tolerate three hours a day of therapy and may do better with a different rehabilitation option. In contrast, someone who is not expected to need extensive rehabilitation may find this much therapy in a hospital setting burdensome. Another consideration is that although these hospitals have elaborate rehabilitation teams, they may not be equipped to handle patients with complicated acute medical problems—say, those who need to be on intravenous antibiotics.

SUBACUTE REHABILITATION HOSPITALIZATION

This is an appropriate option for someone whose recovery is expected to take weeks to months, someone who needs therapy on a daily basis but may not be able to tolerate a full three hours or more each day. It is also a good option for a person who needs a lot of nursing care after surgery, or who may not have someone at home to help physically during the recuperation period. Subacute rehabilitation offers most of the benefits of acute rehabilitation but at a less intensive level. Ancillary services such as on-site x-ray and laboratory facilities may not be available. In addition, although they offer therapy services, subacute centers may not have the full complement of rehabilitation professionals. Beds of this sort are often located on a separate wing or floor of an acute medical hospital, or in a nursing home.

REHABILITATION AT HOME

In this form of rehabilitation, medical professionals come to the patient's home and provide all or most of the necessary care (physical and/or occupational therapy, nursing, and sometimes physician visits). Someone may come in to help with dressing and bathing, cleaning the house, and even doing errands such as grocery shopping.

Home care is typically recommended for someone who is unable to leave home because of temporary or permanent physical constraints. It has become increasingly popular as insurance companies recognize that it is often an economical and nurturing way to provide care.

One limitation of home care is its lack of access to specialized equipment. This may include exercise equipment, pain-controlling modalities such as ultrasound, parallel bars for gait training, or the tools and equipment necessary to fabricate braces. The care that is provided is usually intermittent, so that the patient is without constant medical supervision. In many cases this is appropriate; however, some patients need around-the-clock care.

OUTPATIENT REHABILITATION

Outpatient rehabilitation is ideal for those who are in transition from a hospital setting (either an acute hospital where the surgery was done or a rehabilitation hospital) to their homes or who will no longer be receiving home care. Many people are released shortly after they have surgery and go directly into an outpatient setting. Others go to an outpatient setting after having received another type of rehabilitation first. The appropriate patients generally are ready for a more active type of rehabilitation and are usually able to dress and bathe themselves and move around independently (often with a wheelchair or some other type of assistive device).

The benefits of outpatient rehabilitation include access to specialized equipment and to multiple therapists. The likelihood of finding a therapist experienced in treating polio-related problems is greater than in home care, where assignments are often based on geographic location and scheduling issues.

Among the limitations of outpatient rehabilitation are the frequency and duration of the therapy: appointments typically last thirty to sixty minutes two or three times a week. Patients are often given assignments to do on their own (called a *home exercise program*). Those who follow through on their home exercise program can progress fairly quickly, even if therapy appointments are less frequent than in other settings. The drawback is that a therapist is not available to supervise the program; if the exercises are done incorrectly, progress may be slow.

Regardless of whether someone has had polio, surgery should be approached with forethought and careful planning, except in the most critical life-threatening situations. Polio survivors need not necessarily rule out surgery in the absence of an emergency, but rather should approach it asking, What are the risks? and What are the benefits? If the benefits outweigh the risks and the decision is to undergo an operation, careful planning will likely make the entire process much easier and the chances of a successful outcome much greater.

CHAPTER 22

Complementary and Alternative Medicine

Complementary and alternative medicine (CAM) includes a wide variety of treatments such as acupuncture, massage, and herbal medicines that may or may not be useful to polio survivors. The Office of Alternative Medicine at the National Institutes of Health defines CAM as "a broad domain of healing resources that encompasses all health systems, modalities and practices and their accompanying theories and beliefs, other than those intrinsic to the politically dominant health system of a particular society or culture in a given historical period."[1]

Though many CAM treatments do not have proven value, the use of such therapies is increasing by leaps and bounds. Billions of dollars are spent each year, primarily by patients themselves rather than by insurers. Not surprisingly, a fair amount of controversy surrounds CAM. Some experts in health care argue that the treatments are ineffective, generally unproven, and potentially harmful. Moreover, they correctly contend that the training, licensure, and regulation of CAM practitioners are often inadequate. Opponents further argue that CAM practitioners prey on desperate individuals by offering them little help for large sums of money.

However, CAM has its well-respected proponents in the medical community who counter that traditional medical treatments do not work for everyone, and that CAM offers reasonable complementary, and sometimes alternative, therapies. They contend that individuals suffering from chronic or incurable medical conditions should have other options. For those who believe that the traditional medical community has "failed" them, or who simply want a more "holistic" approach, advocates claim that CAM provides reasonable alternatives. This debate is not likely to be resolved in the near future, so polio survivors (and everyone else) are left wondering whether or not to try CAM.

The philosophy of many physicians (myself included) is a middle-of-the-road approach. It seems reasonable to try both traditional and CAM treatments that are likely to offer the best results with the fewest risks. As with all treatments, consider trying any treatments you can afford that are likely to help and unlikely to harm you. The first part is easy: if you can afford the treatment (or if it is covered by your health insurance plan), then cost is not a barrier. The remainder of the statement requires a little more thought. Because most CAM treatments have not undergone the rigorous scientific testing to which many (but not all) traditional treatments have been subjected, it is often difficult to determine which CAM treatments might be the most helpful with the fewest side effects. In this chapter I comment on some of the more common CAM treatments that polio survivors are seeking out (a more complete list is given in Table 22.1). Keep in mind that any treatments you are considering should be *affordable, helpful, and safe.*

Acupuncture

Medicinal acupuncture dates back to several millennia before the Common Era and is probably the most widely known and most frequently used of the CAM treatments. Proponents of acupuncture

Table 22.1 Categories of complementary and alternative medicine

Category:	Examples:
Manipulative therapies (body work)	Chiropractic, craniosacral therapy, massage, reflexology, shiatsu (acupressure)
Exercise/movement therapies	Tai chi, qong exercise, yoga, Alexander technique, Feldenkrais therapy, Pilates therapy
Physical modalities	Sound (music therapy), light therapy, oxygen therapy, magnetic therapy
Mind-body therapies	Meditation, visualization, guided imagery, biofeedback, hypnosis
Nutritional therapy	Specialized diet, nutritional supplements
Botanical medicine	Herbal therapy
Comprehensive systems of care	Traditional Chinese medicine (TCM), ayurvedic medicine, naturopathic medicine

Note: From J. K. Silver, "Practice Management," *State of the Art Reviews*, 13, No. 1, p. 116, Philadelphia, Harley & Belfus, 1999. Reprinted with permission.

justifiably contend that it has been in existence so long because it works. The basic premise comes from Chinese medicine, in which a *yin* and a *yang* are equally distributed. When an imbalance occurs, disease is thought to be the result. Acupuncture helps to restore the balance.

Acupuncture really describes a family of procedures that stimulate different parts of the body in order to redirect energy flow (Qi). The most common form involves using sterile disposable needles that penetrate the skin at specific locations. Once the needles are in place, they may be gently manipulated by hand or by a machine that generates electrical impulses. Considerable evidence suggests that acupuncture works in part by stimulating the release of opioid peptides, small chemicals produced by the body that can help diminish pain sensations.

Although acupuncture has been touted to work on just about every known illness and medical condition, the truth is that it may be helpful in some circumstances and useless in others. In polio survivors, acupuncture may be useful to control pain—particularly postpolio muscle pain. Acupuncture may also be useful for treating tendinitis and neck and back pain.[2] The concern that acupuncture will mask a serious medical problem is largely unfounded. If such a condition exists (for instance, an undetected cancer that is causing pain), acupuncture will not alleviate the symptoms. It is much more likely that an individual will seek out acupuncture treatment for a prolonged period and simply ignore the fact that it is not working.

My advice to polio survivors with respect to using acupuncture to treat pain is to first meet with your polio doctor and discuss your symptoms and concerns. Follow his or her advice in terms of tests necessary for diagnosis. Consider and preferably try the traditional medical treatments that the doctor suggests. If you continue to have pain that your physician is convinced is not due to a life-threatening or potentially disabling medical condition, then consider trying acupuncture. It is safe when done by a reputable practitioner, but is probably quite costly.

Acupuncture may be helpful in a variety of medical conditions, but should be used as a complement rather than an alternative to traditional medical therapies. Acupuncture may be safely used in conjunction with traditional medicine in almost all circumstances, for instance in treating sinus and respiratory conditions (such as asthma or bronchitis). Acupuncture is not advisable as a treatment for polio-related respiratory problems due to muscle weakness, nor is it useful to treat sleep apnea. Alone or in conjunction with other medical therapies, acupuncture can be useful to treat a variety of addictions including alcohol and tobacco. Anyone who has been unable to stop an addiction through other methods should consider trying acupuncture. Whatever the reason, consult your polio doctor first. Acupuncture is a medical therapy ideally used by polio survivors who are in close communication with the physicians who are overseeing their care.

Magnets

Legitimate evidence suggests that magnets may be effective for treating pain in polio survivors that arises from a variety of medical disorders.[3] How magnets work to alleviate pain is unknown. Also unknown is the proper size of the magnets, the appropriate strength of the magnetic field, and where on the body to place the magnets. As with acupuncture, magnets are thought to be safe to use.

Manual Therapies

For the purposes of this chapter, manual therapies are those that involve healing through physical touch; examples include massage and chiropractic manipulation. Physical and occupational therapists often use manual therapies as well. Numerous studies have shown the benefits of certain types of manual treatments. They can be very soothing and may help injuries to heal. Yet manual therapies that are too aggressive can be extremely dangerous and have been known to lead to severe paralysis.

Polio survivors who are interested in manual therapy to relieve pain should first consult their doctors; if given the go-ahead, they should seek treatment with someone reputable. Gentle manual therapy has an exceedingly low risk of serious injury. Regardless of how "gentle" the treatment, polio survivors should _never_ allow anyone to forcibly manipulate their spines. Owing to muscular weakness and regional or generalized bone loss, even slight spinal manipulation can have catastrophic results in polio survivors. Very gentle sustained cervical traction or gentle massage (muscle energy techniques) involving the muscles around the spine can be quite appropriate, however.

Medicinal Herbs and Other Natural Remedies

A common belief is that medicines derived from herbs and other "natural" products are better than those developed in the laboratory. This may be true for some medications; however, many medicinal herbs and other natural remedies not only provide inadequate solutions for medical conditions but also may be downright dangerous. To understand how natural products may pose a health threat, think of childhood warnings not to eat mushrooms: although the majority of mushrooms are perfectly safe to eat and even quite nutritious, some are deadly. Obviously, it is exceedingly unlikely that anyone would market a known poisonous herb (or mushroom), but the natural remedies that are available without a prescription may not have undergone the rigorous testing and licensing procedures required of prescription drugs. Moreover, natural herbs combined with prescription medications, or even other natural herbs, may prove to be a dangerous combination. For example, the herbal remedy ginkgo combined with the prescription drug coumadin may be fatal because of the blood-thinning (anticoagulant) properties of both.

Once again, it is best to talk to your doctor if you are considering any natural remedies. Be aware, however, that your doctor may not know much about a nonprescription medicinal herb. Not many scientific studies have been made of these products, besides which medical schools do not generally teach physicians about such treatments. It may be frustrating for patients who want to consult their doctors about natural remedies, but they may not be able to provide the same knowledgeable advice that they can for more traditional treatments. Remember that there are literally thousands of CAM treatment options, and that information about their efficacy and risks may be lacking. As CAM therapies become more popular and are better studied, more information will surely be available.

In summary, CAM treatments may offer polio survivors complementary or alternative therapy options, but they should be *safe, helpful, and affordable.* In the future more proven CAM treatments may be available, but some CAM treatments may fall out of favor because they are deemed ineffective or dangerous. If you are considering CAM treatments, check with your doctor first!

CHAPTER 23

Designing a Safe and Comfortable Living Environment

An environment that is comfortable, safe, and convenient is important to everyone. The environment of polio survivors should allow them also to conserve energy and to be as independent as possible. Creating an environment where polio survivors can thrive takes careful thought, and consideration of each individual's specific needs.

Before becoming discouraged about the potential cost to improve your environment, remember that it will cost you nothing now to continue reading. This chapter will propose ways in which you can economically change your environment and resources where you may be able to find financial support. Consider the following questions: Are you able to move about your home completely independently, without fatigue or fear of falling? Do you avoid going to certain locations (even within your own home) because they are not accessible or because they are simply too much trouble? Are you concerned about not being able to continue your current vocation? Would you enjoy it if physical barriers were removed and you could go where you wanted, at your leisure? Would you feel better if you had more energy and could move about more easily? Would you feel more independent if you could operate appliances without asking for help with small, hard-to-reach controls? This chapter provides a starting point for addressing these quality-of-life issues.

Making Modifications and Finding Help

Trying to decide what kind of modifications to your environment will be most beneficial takes time and careful planning. Think about whether it would be easier and more cost efficient to move into an updated, accessible dwelling rather than perform extensive modifications to your current home. Workplaces are generally more difficult for individuals to modify, but one can usually take a number of simple steps to make the work environment safer and easier to use.

Before making any decisions about what you want to do, consider getting some professional help. Architects and contractors who specialize in building or modifying homes for persons with disabilities will generally meet with you and offer suggestions at no cost or a minimal fee (depending on the extent of the advice you are seeking and whether you ultimately hire them to do the work). Be wary of individuals who advertise that they are experts in modifications for persons with disabilities. Some of them may be—but not all. Ask for the names and phone numbers of satisfied customers, and either go to see the work they have done for others or ask for photos.

For genuinely helpful and unbiased advice, ask your doctor to set up a home visit with a physical or occupational therapist who has expertise in recommending home modifications (the cost of this consultation may be paid by your health-insurance provider). Large rehabilitation hospitals also may have an assistive technology department that is devoted to keeping up on the latest technological advances for individuals with disabilities. A consultation with these

Table 23.1 Resources for financial assistance for home/work modifications

Your state division of vocational rehabilitation
Local, state, and federal housing agencies
Veterans Administration
Administration on Aging
Medicare/Medicaid
Nonprofit consumer, advocacy, and civic groups
Local post-polio support groups

Note: Available resources will vary depending on the group or agency, the geographic location, and the individual's specific needs and qualifications.

health professionals (ordered by your doctor) can be extremely valuable and again may be covered by your health-insurance provider. While gathering information, check books and other resources available from local, state, and federal agencies, senior and disability advocacy groups, and professional publishers devoted to disability issues.

Financial Resources

If you are able to afford to make modifications to your existing home or workplace, then you are fortunate indeed. However, if the modifications you desperately need are out of your price range, consider some of the suggestions in Table 23.1 for securing the requisite money.

Various local, state, and federal agencies assist disabled and/or elderly individuals with financing of new homes or modifications of existing homes. Nonprofit consumer, advocacy, and civic groups also are valuable resources. Examples include Habitat for Humanity; the Rotary, Shriner, and Lions clubs; and churches, synagogues, and other religious organizations. Post-polio support groups may also provide loans and grants to polio survivors in particular.[1] Some banks also provide low-interest loans for purchasing assistive technology or financing home modifications. In budgeting your costs, factor in deductions allowable by the IRS. In general, special equipment purchased for medical reasons can be deducted. Of course, it is vital to maintain accurate records. Thus, keep all sales receipts and ask your doctor to send you a *letter of medical necessity* to keep in your files for any big-ticket items. You might also check with an accountant to be sure that you are in compliance with IRS guidelines.

Modifications—An Overview

The modifications suggested in this chapter are meant to accomplish the following:

1. Create an environment in which you can move about easily and with minimal effort. This decreases energy expenditure and generally makes it more enjoyable to do what you need or want to do.
2. Make your environment safe, in order to reduce the risk of falling and sustaining a serious injury.

In order to accomplish these goals, you need to recognize the fact that a lot of small tasks and inconveniences sap your energy and strength. Therefore, the only way to genuinely improve your environment is to look carefully at individual pieces and see how they impact the total picture. Small changes can make a large difference in terms of improving mobility, decreasing energy expenditure, and ensuring safety.

The suggestions in this chapter are just that—suggestions. Not everything will work for everyone. The ideas presented here are simply meant to encourage polio survivors to explore options that will make the environments in which they live easier to navigate. Integrating the material presented here with that in Chapters 14 and 16 is essential.

General Home Tips

The "ideal home" is different for everyone. Traditionally, homes that have been modified to accommodate individuals with disabilities have been criticized for resembling a hospital environment. The focus of this chapter is on how to utilize many different options that may or may not be specifically designed for persons with disabilities. The environment in which we all work and live is becoming ever more technologically advanced. Everyone has opportunities to get more done with less effort. Improving the environment of polio survivors may simply mean taking advantage of some of the latest consumer products that are widely available to the general public.

One of the suggestions that I routinely make to everyone, regardless of age or medical history, is to sit while showering. Polio survivors expend unnecessary energy by standing to bathe, when they could be sitting. Moreover, showers are notorious as the site of many falls. Because we are all creatures of habit, when I suggest to polio survivors that they may want to consider sitting down to shower, I often meet a great deal of resistance. The following are the most frequent responses I hear: (1) I take very short showers, so I don't need to sit; (2) I have always stood in the shower and don't think I could change; and (3) I have never fallen in the shower, so why should I change?

My response is always the same, "If it is very important to you to stand in the shower, then continue to do so. However, if standing while showering is not something that truly gives you pleasure, consider sitting down." I give the example of my eight-year-old son, who has always sat in the shower, because all of the homes built in our neighborhood had showers with seats. (In our area, the current trend in construction is to install showers with seats, since the cost is not much more than a traditional stall, and the seat adds a level of convenience for the home owner.) Although there is no reason for my son to sit, he finds it relaxing after a long day of running around and playing with his friends. If I were to ask him whether he realized that some people stand during their entire shower, he would probably look at me with a quizzical expression and assume I was talking about days long gone.

My point is that many items are designed to make us more comfortable and allow us to relax and conserve energy. Polio survivors should carefully consider what options are available, not reject them out of hand because they are new or different. Admittedly, sitting down to bathe will conserve only a small amount of energy, but keep in mind that a cumulative effect accrues as one modifies one's environment in a variety of ways.

When you begin to consider modifying or customizing your home, you will need to start with the basics.[2] How wide should the doors be? Where should the electrical outlets and light switches be so that you can reach them easily? How will the layout of the rooms affect their accessibility? Should you install an elevator or a stair lift to go from one level to the next? The answer to these and other questions will vary depending on whether you are ambulatory or use a wheelchair or scooter. Doorways should be wide enough to allow you to pass through easily. Rooms should be large enough (and uncluttered enough) for you to move about and change directions without difficulty. Electrical sockets and light switches should be at a level that allows you to operate them without bending, stooping, or reaching overhead. Toggle or rocker light switches turn on and off easily. Lights with dimmers allow you to control the amount of light without using multiple lamps or overhead lights. Lever door handles may be easier to use than traditional doorknobs. Environmental control units allow you to perform multiple functions (such as turning on and off the television, radio, and lights, locking and unlocking the door, signaling to someone in another room). Stair lifts are ideal for individuals who live in multilevel homes and are at risk of falling. Although they can be a costly modification, they may be much more economical than moving.

There is no one formula that works for everyone. Therefore, taking time to consider what will help you most and seeking advice from professionals during the planning stages is crucial.

ENTRANCES AND EXITS

Entrances and exits should be easily accessible and safe to use. In poor weather conditions, a carport and covered walkway, or a door connecting the garage to your home or office, is ideal. Ground surfaces should be gently sloped to allow drainage; a ramp may be necessary as well. In general, for a motorized wheelchair or scooter a 1-foot rise requires 12 feet of length. Therefore, if the building you want to enter is 3 feet above ground level, you will need a 36-foot ramp. All stairs should be outfitted with at least one railing that is sturdy and secure (sometimes a railing on both sides is advantageous). A level paved surface leading to the mailbox, garden, or patio is preferable. Hand-held door openers to the garage or car are easy to operate and readily available.

KITCHEN BASICS

Kitchens are the sites of many injuries due to burns, falls, wounds from sharp cutting utensils, and so forth. Despite the fact that kitchens pose some hazards, they are often the focal point of a home, where individuals spend a lot of time and take pleasure in cooking and conversing with friends and family members. Therefore making the kitchen safe, convenient, and comfortable is a priority.

The first question is how much maneuverable space is there in the kitchen? Could the floor plan be rearranged to allow easier access to the cooking, eating, and dishwashing areas? Next, consider the storage areas. Cupboards and drawers should be at a level that is accessible and does not involve reaching or stooping. Some built-in work surfaces have generous counter overhangs that allow someone to pull up a wheelchair and sit down to work. Pull-out shelves and counters allow more usable space when necessary and can be put away when not needed. Sinks and grills that have an opening underneath are ideal places to do chores while sitting. A note of caution: working over a hot surface requires extreme care and may be hazardous while sitting if one cannot get out of the way of hot spilled food.

Appliances vary greatly, but consider purchasing those with self-cleaning features (a self-cleaning oven or a freezer that does not require defrosting). Side-by-side refrigerator/freezer combinations are generally easier to access than the top-and-bottom models. Electric stoves are safer than gas because they have no open flame. Staggering the burners helps to avoid getting burned when reaching to a back burner. Remember that burner controls on the front of the stove are easy to get at and eliminate the need for reaching over the burners, but they are also easier for children to turn on. A mirror installed over the stove allows continuous observation of the back burners without stretching to check them. Wall-type ovens situated at eye level are ideal for baking.

BATHROOM BASICS

Bathrooms are another site of many serious injuries, owing to the slippery and hard surfaces. Therefore, the main goals for the bathroom are safety and utility. The first consideration is the layout and floor plan. With accessibility usually an issue, if the bathroom is too small it may be necessary to build a larger bathroom or to convert an existing room into a bathroom. Bathrooms are notorious for having unexpected accessibility problems, so be certain before you start that there is enough room to enter, exit, and turn around once inside with a wheelchair. If you are not using a wheelchair now but are in the process of designing a bathroom, think about making it large enough to accommodate a wheelchair in the future. Even if *you* do not need the extra space, someone else might.

Next consider the sink space. Ideally the sink should allow polio survivors to sit down for grooming (regardless of whether or not they use a wheelchair). Grooming is time consuming, and sitting to groom is an easy way to conserve energy and prevent muscular fatigue that may lead to falling and sustaining a serious injury or permanent loss of strength due to overuse. Faucets should be within easy reach (long handles and levers are easy to use) and a mirror should be placed at your eye level while sitting. Light switches, outlets, towel racks, and soap dishes should all be easily accessible.

All toilets should have professionally installed grab bars (not towel racks!) to assist in getting on and off. Raised toilet seats also decrease the amount of effort required. Wall-mounted toilets allow wheelchairs to maneuver close to the seat without hitting the base, thereby helping with transfers from the wheelchair to the commode.

Bathtubs and showers are inherently dangerous because of their hard, slippery surfaces; therefore, creating a safe bathing environment is essential. Fortunately, a number of modifications can greatly diminish the risk of falls while bathing. Examples are tub benches and shower seats, which also provide relief for legs that are susceptible to overuse while standing. Grab bars can be strategically placed in order to help with balance and transfers. A hand-held faucet (shower or bath) can be useful in order to get at hard-to-reach places without straining. For individuals who need additional help getting in and out of the bath, several models of lifts are available. Tub and shower floor surfaces should be level and covered with a skid-resistant surface.

Office Basics

Creating a safe and productive office environment pays huge dividends in increasing efficiency, decreasing fatigue, and improving one's overall quality of work. Employers' interest in office efficiency has created a demand for inexpensive equipment that allows many of us to do our jobs more easily. Despite the fact that much of this equipment is not specifically designed for individuals with disabilities, it is readily available and easily adaptable for polio survivors. How much and what kind depends on the specifics of any given job. However, general guidelines specifically addressing "desk jobs" may be helpful both at the work site and in a home office.

In order to design an efficient and productive work space, first consider seating. The ideal chair is comfortable and adjustable, with a sturdy back support and armrests. Your feet should rest firmly on the ground, or on a footstool if necessary. (Footstools are not ideal, because one can trip and fall over them.) Both the chair and the desk should be conveniently located in order to minimize the number of times getting up and down is necessary.

Next, evaluate the work surface. It should be at a comfortable height for reading, writing, computer use, and the like. Equipment that is readily available at office supply stores (and may help with posture and with decreasing arm and neck fatigue) includes forearm rests (also called data arms), book stands, slanted writing boards, computer copy stands (document holders to keep papers at eye level), and telephone headsets or speaker phones.

For those who are avid computer users, voice-activated word-processing software has improved dramatically. People who take the time to learn to use this software may find it to be a lifesaver.

Community and Long-Distance Travel

The concept of *universal design* simply means that the environment is designed so that all people, regardless of whether they have a disability or not, can move about freely without adaptation. This is an ideal environment, and as most polio survivors can attest, one that seldom exists. In order to navigate in the community and during long-distance travel, it helps to be prepared for barriers and unexpected obstacles.

One of the first decisions is how to travel. The mode will vary depending on a polio survivor's strength, mobility, and preferences. Regardless of whether an individual walks, uses a wheelchair or scooter, or drives, some basic tips may make the journey easier and more enjoyable by reducing pain, fatigue, and potential overuse of the muscles.

For travel by car, consider hand controls and cruise control. Both options are useful for individuals with significant leg weakness. Remember that driving involves extensive muscular contractions for prolonged periods and can result in significant overuse of the muscles. Hand controls are not for everyone; however, for polio survivors they may significantly reduce fatigue and overuse of the legs. Cruise control is a nice feature for anyone who drives on highways or freeways. Handicapped parking plates or placards allow polio survivors to park near their destination. Handicapped parking permits can be obtained at the local registry of motor vehicles and generally involve filling out a form and obtaining a doctor's signature.

Assistive Technology

The field of assistive technology is rapidly developing and is focused on providing individuals who have a disability with products that maximize their ability to function. These items may be available commercially or custom designed for the user.[3]

The assistive technology department in the hospital where I work is staffed by physical, occupational, and speech therapists who have extensive knowledge of the latest products. I refer people to this department for a variety of reasons. Sometimes they want to learn to use voice-activated computer software, or they want units that permit the control of appliances by a simple switch or a voice command. Polio survivors may want a hand-held device that allows them to control the room thermostat, lighting, television, and radio—or to lock and unlock the door that accesses the home.

The field of assistive technology is rapidly expanding and changing. Probably the best way to learn more is to go to a large rehabilitation hospital in your area that has an assistive technology department. As noted earlier, an evaluation there may be covered by your medical insurance (although the products may not be).

CHAPTER 24

Insurance and Disability Benefits

During the polio epidemics in the first half of the twentieth century, health insurance was uncommon. Many individuals who became ill with polio relied on small "polio policies" (insurance policies that specifically covered the care of an individual who contracted polio) or financial support from the National Foundation for Infantile Paralysis. Others simply did not seek treatment or paid for it themselves. Today, decades later, health insurance is something that most of us rely on to cover the majority of our medical bills. Debating how medical resources should be allocated and who should pay for these resources is the topic of many books and will not be addressed here. Rather, the following suggestions are meant to be a useful guide in navigating the health-insurance maze—regardless of whether you have managed care or some other type of insurance coverage.

The health-care industry is in constant flux. What is available today in terms of health insurance may be defunct tomorrow. Nevertheless, whether the insurance is funded by the government, by an employer, or paid for privately, some simple guidelines may be helpful.

1. When you are choosing health insurance, always assume that if you pay less, you get less—no matter what the brochures or the

company representatives tell you. Health-care is a business and works on the same principles as any industry. If you buy a Volkswagen, you don't get to take the Mercedes home.

2. When you are reviewing the benefits package, check to see what channels you have to go through to get those benefits. For instance, if the health plan you are considering offers unlimited physical therapy visits, determine what approval process is needed in order to have those visits covered. Often the benefits appear to be unlimited, but in reality someone behind the scenes is in charge of approving the visits.

3. If you need referrals in order to go to specialists, think about the process of getting these referrals from your doctor. If you are having difficulty, you should consider changing doctors or changing health-insurance plans. Some are so restrictive that even an accommodating physician cannot get the health insurer to pay for services. Keep in mind that you are one of many individuals for whom your doctor may need to "go to bat," and even willing doctors get worn down by the process. Changing to a plan that is less restrictive may be the easiest (and sometimes the only) way to get what you need.

4. Don't let little perquisites sway you. Many plans offer perks to get you to switch insurers. These perks are often very inexpensive compared to other benefits that the companies limit or do not cover at all. For instance, one common perk that initially sounds appealing is coverage for eyeglasses. Although prescription eyeglasses can be expensive, they are far cheaper than rehabilitation services. Keep in mind that *one* physical therapy visit often will cost more than prescription eyeglasses. Health insurers are smart enough to know that if they can get people to sign on for small (but enticing) perks and limit the costly rehabilitation benefits (that polio survivors often desperately need), then they can make money.

5. Carefully review all of the rehabilitation benefits, including physical, occupational, and speech therapy—inpatient, outpatient,

and home services. Are there limits on therapy services? Are therapy services covered only in certain facilities? Check what is covered in terms of bracing and orthotics (often listed as durable medical equipment or hardware). Review the coverage for acute and subacute rehabilitation hospital services; these are critical for polio survivors.

6. Last but not least, be sure you will have access to a knowledgeable polio doctor and to other specialists (e.g., pulmonologists, orthopedists) whose services you may need at some point.

Disability and Work

By and large, polio survivors are determined, energetic, and industrious. So when individuals face increasing disability due to Post-Polio Syndrome or other health problems, the decision to choose an alternative career path or to discontinue working altogether is not made easily. Sunny Roller, a polio survivor, writes: "When we who had polio were growing up, our physicians didn't know enough about polio's late effects to warn us about our career choices. We chose our professions and vocations based on our interests and levels of disability at the time. Many of us never imagined that we'd need to adapt to the changing labor market trends *and* to the alarming effects of polio as we approached the pinnacles of our chosen careers. We weren't prepared with 'an alternate plan B.' "[1]

Unfortunately, as Roller writes, many polio survivors have to face difficult decisions just as they are at the pinnacle of their chosen careers. In some instances they are able to continue their current jobs, albeit with modifications. For a college professor, a reduced classroom workload and a voice-activated word-processing system for paperwork may do the trick. For a bridge inspector, avoiding climbing and lifting heavy objects may be enough. For a nurse, switching from the hospital wards to an administrative position may work. For a grocery produce supervisor who travels from store to store by car, assigning the construction of displays to less senior employees and getting hand controls for the car could make the job manageable. The list is endless.

Modifying jobs, however, is often easier said than done. Employers who are unwilling to be accommodating can easily thwart attempts by polio survivors to change their work situation in order to continue in the same or a similar position. What if the college professor's employer refuses to agree to a reduced classroom teaching schedule, or the bridge inspector is required to climb ladders and lift heavy objects or face being fired? What if the produce supervisor has no junior employees to help build displays, or the nurse is unable to find an administrative position? Despite the good intentions of the Americans with Disabilities Act (ADA) signed in 1990, the reality is that it mandates only "reasonable accommodations." Individuals with disabilities who have had uncooperative employers can attest to the fact that this law is often not enforceable, and even when it is, may involve thousands of dollars in legal fees and years of waiting for the court system to work. The concept of reasonable accommodations is so subjective than an uncooperative employer may ultimately prevail—even if the case finally makes it to court.

Some polio survivors may find that their work situation is unmanageable even if their employers are willing to make any and all accommodations necessary to keep valued employees. For instance, in the examples above the individuals may simply not be able to work the number of hours required, owing to fatigue. Their commute may be too long, or they may be in so much pain that they are not able to do their job effectively. In such situations, it may be mandatory that a polio survivor give up his or her current position or face increasing disability and/or being fired or forced to resign. The decision then is between retiring and finding a less demanding occupation.

Anyone who has changed from one vocation to another knows that the initial decision and transition are the most difficult. Yet some polio survivors may find a relatively easy way to move to another profession. For instance, a college professor who has spent a lifetime teaching may choose to do some freelance writing, tutoring, or teach occasional adult-education courses. A bridge inspector may be able to do some part-time consulting work in an office setting. Although these would likely not be equivalent in terms of compensation, they might be alternatives worth pursuing in order to remain active and to achieve some degree of financial support. Moreover, there is always the opportunity for someone to learn an entirely new skill. Instead of the bridge inspector's turning to consulting work, he may want to learn about how computers operate and find a job providing technical support by phone to computer users.

Disabled individuals who are interested in vocational counseling and possible retraining can contact their state's vocational rehabilitation division. Vocational rehabilitation is jointly funded by the federal and state governments, and the offices are generally listed in the telephone book under *state government services.* After an orientation and evaluation, these agencies will provide vocational counseling and often will pay for the courses and equipment needed so that disabled individuals can work at an alternative vocation. On-the-job training and on-the-job assistance may also be provided. As with any government agency, the process may be time-consuming, but it can be well worth the effort.

For polio survivors who are unable to continue working to support themselves financially, one possibility is to apply for Social Security benefits. That decision, although heart wrenching, is a viable (and sometimes the most reasonable) option for polio survivors. It requires support from a treating physician who can substantiate the diagnosis and subsequent disability of the individual who is applying, and the process can be long and laborious. For those polio sur-vivos who are unable to continue working, Social Security benefits are usually granted (although not necessarily on the first attempt)—as they should be.

Rosemary Marx, a nurse who has PPS, describes what it was like for her when she applied for Social Security benefits after she could no longer work in her chosen profession. "I was denied benefits twice. In order to get my benefits, I had to hire an attorney and appear before a judge. That was a very stressful time for me. I was already feeling guilty about not working, and I was having a lot of pain. I felt like I had to beg for help." It took Rosemary a total of ten months from the time she initially applied to get approval for the benefits. When she finally was approved, she had mixed emotions. "Though I was greatly relieved to get the benefits, the fact that I had a written document confirming that I was permanently disabled was very depressing for me. For the first time, I had a good cry."[2]

SOCIAL SECURITY DISABILITY BENEFITS

Federal government disability programs fall into two general categories. The first is *Social Security Disability Insurance* (SSDI). In order to qualify for SSDI, individuals need to be disabled and to have an employment history whereby they have developed work credits and contributed to the FICA taxes through which SSDI is funded. Substantial documentation is required both from the applicant and from a physician who can substantiate the individual's claim of total permanent disability (federal programs do not cover partial or short-term disability). This documentation from a physician is critical.

Joe Carson is a fifty-five-year-old polio survivor who worked more than twenty years for the same company as manager of a record store. In his late forties he developed PPS and began losing strength in his legs. He started to fall routinely, often in front of customers at the store. Joe also had severe fatigue, which caused him to have difficulty doing paperwork—particularly in the afternoon. When Joe went to his polio doctor, the physician agreed that Joe had PPS but did not support Joe's decision to file for disability. Unfortunately, Joe was unable to continue in his demanding job and was demoted with a substantial pay cut. He changed doctors, and the new doctor supported Joe's decision to go on disability. Joe is fortunate in that he had private (commercial) disability insurance and also was eligible for SSDI. However, Joe's private insurance was based on 80 percent of his salary; the fact that he had been forced to work at a lower salary affected the amount of money he receives on a monthly basis now that he is no longer working.

This example illustrates how important it is to have a doctor involved who understands polio and PPS, and who is sympathetic and knowledgeable with respect to disability issues. However, no doctor should consider every polio survivor an automatic candidate for disability benefits. Many factors must be weighed, including the individual's current and predicted health status and the demands of the job in question. For any given person other factors may be involved, such as the length of the commute to work, the presence of another adult who is contributing financially to the household, and so on. For instance, if a polio survivor lives with his wife, who is able to support both of them financially, then part-time work for him might be a better option than discontinuing work altogether. But if he has no other means of financial support, part-time work may not provide sufficient income. These are all considerations that polio survivors and their doctors need to discuss prior to formally filing for disability benefits.

The second federal program is *Social Security Income* (SSI), which is funded through general tax funds. This program is similar to SSDI in that one needs to prove disability (by providing copies of

Table 24.1 Documents needed to apply for SSDI

Medical history (including a description of the original polio, new limitations,
current level of function, and diagnosis of Post-Polio Syndrome)
Social Security card or record of the number
Proof of age
Proof of work history for the past fifteen years (including names and addresses
of employers)
Proof of income (including W-2s or federal tax returns)

---

medical records and sometimes undergoing a physical examination at the request of the agency). Unlike SSDI, there is no work credit requirement; instead, an individual must show financial need in the form of limited income and resources.

As in the case of Rosemary Marx, benefits are often not granted on the first request. There is an appeals process, which may take several months to navigate. An attorney skilled in disability issues may be helpful. Having been the physician who performs a physical examination on individuals applying for various disability benefits, I have found that the majority of people who are truly disabled but are denied benefits simply do not prepare adequately for the process. Providing information that substantiates a claim of disability is imperative. Successful applicants prepare thoroughly and provide credible and complete documentation to support their claim. Table 24.1 lists the information you need to gather to apply for SSDI. The Social Security toll-free information phone number is (800) 772-1213.

OTHER DISABILITY BENEFIT OPTIONS

The federally funded government programs are only available to individuals who are totally and permanently disabled. Commercially available disability policies, purchased either privately or by employers, vary greatly. Many cover short-term or partial disability.

Any polio survivor who has this type of policy should carefully review it in order to determine what benefits are offered.

Some states have disability insurance programs as well. Generally they are funded by employees who contribute a portion of the premium through payroll deductions. Benefits are allocated depending on the amount contributed to the fund.

Navigating health-insurance and disability-insurance issues is never easy. Even skilled attorneys and individuals in the health-care industry are frequently confused by changing regulations and rules. It is impossible to understand every detail of these different insurances; the goal is to obtain whatever benefits a specific individual needs. To do so, one needs the assistance of a competent doctor who can help to direct care and document disability status if necessary. One may also need to hire an attorney who specializes in disability-related issues. Polio survivors will perhaps want to check with their local support groups for advice and information specific to their geographic region.

CHAPTER 25

Sex and Intimacy

I am rarely surprised by the things people tell me during an office visit; however, not long ago I had the privilege of treating a polio survivor who had a number of serious medical issues. His list of problems was so long and overwhelming that I did what I often do in order to have a place to start. I asked him, "What is the one thing I can do to help you the most?" I expected him to reply that he wanted me to help him keep walking, or that his pain was intolerable and he needed relief, or even that he wanted me to help him continue working in the construction job he was becoming unable to manage. Instead he replied, "I want you to help me with my sex life." Here was a man on the verge of losing his job, who could barely walk and was in such severe discomfort that nearly every movement contorted his face in pain. How could it be that what he wanted most was to have a better sex life? It was a wake-up call for me. I learned then and there that I needed to make the topic of sexual functioning and intimacy a priority in people who were having problems and came to me seeking medical advice.

For health-care providers, broaching the topic of sexual functioning and intimacy can be akin to walking on a surface hidden with land mines. For some people, asking about their sex life is a welcome invitation, and for others it is a rude invasion of their privacy. After several encounters such as the one described above, I began to think about intimacy and sexual relations in polio survivors. I wondered how many individuals needed medical advice but had not had the opportunity to ask, or were simply too embarrassed? How did Post-Polio Syndrome affect polio survivors' ability to be physically intimate?

I also wondered how I and other health-care providers could address these important topics with individual patients. How should we broach the subject? Where is the line between giving medical advice and invading an individual's privacy? What advice and treatment could we offer that would be helpful? Since the time that I initially began exploring these issues, I have conducted some research on the topic of physical intimacy in polio survivors. Additionally, I have made this area a formal part of the polio program at our clinic. Throughout this process I have tried to be respectful of a person's privacy and only intervene when I was given permission.

Dispelling Sexual Myths and Stereotypes

For the purposes of this chapter, the terms *sex* and *sexual relations* will be specifically used to describe genital contact, and the term *intimacy* will be used more generally to describe all levels of a physical relationship between two consenting adults. In other settings intimacy may describe an emotional bond between two people, but here it will apply to a physical relationship with another person.

When I decided to include intimacy and sexual relations in this book, I realized that it is a difficult subject for many reasons. First, many find the topic uncomfortable to discuss or read about. Second, myths and stereotypes are so pervasive that they may unduly discourage people from reading this chapter. Third, little research has been published on sexuality and aging in polio survivors. Yet I know from my own clinical practice that many polio survivors have questions and concerns in this area.

One of the most pervasive myths, which marginalizes individuals as they age, is the notion that as people get older they become disengaged from sex. This is simply not true of most people. Studies show that sex continues to play a major role in the lives of people as they age—even into their seventies, eighties, and nineties.[1] The myth arises in part because of long-standing stereotypes of women who become "disinterested" in sex after menopause, and "dirty old men" who continue to be interested in sex as they age. For some people the desire for intimacy and sexual relations may change or even diminish as they age, but for many others that desire remains an important part of their lives. The myths and stereotypes serve no useful purpose and may in fact be harmful to those who desire intimacy but feel ashamed of their yearnings.

Charlotte Eliopoulos, an authority on sexuality and aging, gives some insight into how these myths have been perpetuated. "For many years, sex was a major conversational taboo in our country. Discussion and education concerning this natural, normal process were discouraged and avoided in most circles. Literature on the subject was minimal and usually secured under lock and key. An interest in sex was considered sinful and highly improper . . . The reluctance to accept and intelligently confront human sexuality led to the propagation of numerous myths, the persistence of ignorance and prejudice, and the relegation of sex to a vulgar status."[2]

Encouraging people to accept physical intimacy as an acceptable and even vital part of aging, regardless of whether they have a disability, is beneficial. Those who are loved and generously reciprocate that love on a physically intimate level add an immeasurable richness to their lives—and to the lives of their partners.

The Effects of Illness and Aging

Many medical conditions can impact sexual function in both men and women.[3] Table 25.1 lists some of the more common illnesses and their possible effects. Sometimes even more disabling than the effects of the disease itself are the psychological effects of a chronic disease on one's interest and motivation for continuing to lead a life that includes physical intimacy with a loved one. I do not mean to belittle the real effect that many illnesses have on sexual function, but rather to point out that the daily fight against any chronic disease may become so physically and emotionally draining that interest in intimacy may wane. Often when people say "I want to have sex," what they really mean is that they wish they had the desire and energy to have sex. Occasionally people with chronic illnesses are so consumed with their condition that they use all their energy to combat illness (going to different physicians, trying multiple treatments, and so on). In no way do I suggest that seeking state-of-the-art medical care should be discarded at any point when someone has an illness; however, concentrating on quality-of-life issues—regardless of one's state of health—is essential to fighting any illness. These issues may or may not involve intimacy for any given person. I mean simply to encourage people to take the time to address the topic of intimacy if it is important to them and enhances their quality of life.

MEDICATIONS AND THEIR EFFECTS

Many medications can alter sexual functioning in one way or another.[4] Some of the side effects can be to decrease sexual desire or libido, cause difficulty sustaining an erection (impotence), or have the opposite effect and cause a sustained painful erection (priapism) or painful intercourse (dyspareunia). Table 25.2 lists some common medications which may have side effects that affect physical inti-

Table 25.1 Physical conditions that may interfere with sexual function

---

Men
Arteriosclerosis
Parkinson's disease
Prostate problems
Spine conditions that affect the spinal cord or terminal nerve roots

Women
Decreased level of estrogen
Prolapsed uterus

Both Men and Women
Alcoholism
Arthritis
Bowel or urinary incontinence
Cardiovascular disease
Dementia
Depression
Diabetes
Hypertension
Infections of the genitalia
Multiple sclerosis
Respiratory disease
Stroke
Thyroid problems

---

macy. Regardless of the medication, its benefits should always be weighed against its side effects. Even if a medication potentially affects sexual functioning, it may still be worth taking. Any changes in medication or discontinuation of a medication should be discussed in advance with the prescribing physician.

THE EFFECTS OF NORMAL AGING

Normal aging produces physical changes that are apparent in everyone. We all have an image of how we think we look, which is probably

Table 25.2 Drugs that may be associated with sexual dysfunction (partial list)

Alcohol	Hydralazine
Amphetamines	Hydroxyzine
Antiandrogens	Imipramine
Antihistamines	Lithium carbonate
Atropine	Marijuana
Baclofen	Methantheline bromide
Barbiturates	Methaqualone
Benztropine	Methyldopa
Chlordiazepoxide	Monoamine oxidase inhibitors
Chlorprothixene	Morphine
Cimetidine	Nicotine
Clofibrate	Phenothiazines
Clonidine	Phenoxybenzamine
Cocaine	Phentolamine
Cyclobenzaprine	Propanolol
Dantrolene sodium	Psychedelics (e.g., LSD)
Digitalis	Reserpine
Diazepam	Spironolactone
Dimenhydrinate	Thiazide diuretics
Diphenhydramine	Thioridazine
Guanethidine	Trihexyphenidyl
Heroin	

close to (but not the same as) how we appear to others. This image has changed and evolved over time as we progress from childhood through adolescence and into adulthood. Although the changes our bodies undergo as an adult are more subtle and occur over a much longer period than when we were teenagers, they nevertheless affect our bodies and the images we possess of ourselves.

Some of the normal changes that occur with growing older include alterations in the color and texture of our skin, which appear as wrinkles and age spots. Our hair may be lost or turn shades of gray. Many people have changes in the color of their tooth enamel;

they may lose some or all of their teeth. Weight gain or loss may be a factor. These inevitable physical changes may significantly alter our appearance and can potentially undermine our self-confidence. We live in a society that places extraordinary value on youth and physical perfection, and it is sometimes difficult for all of us to reconcile society's attitudes and prejudices with our own tentative feelings of attractiveness and self-worth. We need to recognize that a poor self-image may directly impact someone's willingness to become physically intimate because they feel awkward and unattractive.

In polio survivors, feelings of attractiveness may also be affected by physical evidence of having had polio (such as muscle atrophy). Individuals may feel awkward if their legs are swollen, discolored, or asymmetric. A brace or a mobility device may cause them to feel less attractive. Clearly, body image affects some people more than others, and there is no right or wrong way to feel.

OTHER FACTORS

Physical intimacy is a complicated topic, subject to many influences and social mores. Some of the issues as one ages are purely physical. For instance, women may have less vaginal lubrication, which can lead to dyspareunia. Men may have difficulty achieving or sustaining an erection. These issues should be brought to the attention of a trusted health-care provider who may be able to offer advice and appropriate medical treatment (which may be as simple as using K-Y jelly for vaginal lubrication, or a medication to treat male impotence).

Another issue that may affect physical intimacy is a lack of privacy. Living situations may be such that privacy is not readily available. Often the solution is simply to make others aware that privacy is desired; a detailed explanation is not necessary. Unfortunately, this is easier said than done. The lack of a partner may also be a barrier to physical intimacy, particularly for women, who tend to live longer than their male counterparts. Regardless of age or gender, individuals may find themselves alone (sometimes by choice) and without the opportunity to be physically intimate.

Disabled persons may encounter additional barriers. For instance, girls who are either born with or acquire a disability are often raised by protective parents who shelter them from men. They may not have opportunities for the normal adolescent rites of passage such as kissing, holding hands, and the like. They may have missed out on sex education because it was often taught during gym class, and many children with disabilities did not take gym.

It is frequently assumed that someone who is disabled is also asexual. This attitude may be born of simple ignorance; however, it can significantly impact the ability to cope with intimacy later in life. As sexuality expert Karen Hwang points out, disabled girls often hear, "No one is going to marry them anyway . . . As a result of this lack of preparation as well as the devastating blows to self-esteem that such repeated messages can deliver, girls with disabilities also tend to be at greater risk physically and psychologically to abuse." Certainly a history of physical or psychological abuse can be a strong barrier to the ability and desire of a woman (or man) to form intimate relationships. But even without experiencing abuse, the stigma of being disabled and therefore "asexual" may haunt many disabled individuals and keep them from participating in physical intimacy.[5]

Abuse and Its Effects

The abuse of some polio survivors is well documented and has taken many forms. In a chilling passage in his autobiography, titled *Black*

Bird Fly Away, polio survivor Hugh Gallagher describes what happened to him when he was hospitalized and paralyzed during his initial polio. "I was raped at some point during the week. I was forcibly violated in a particularly horrible and humiliating manner."[6] Gallagher goes on to describe how a nurse who was caring for him forcibly removed fecal material from his bowels "without warning and without explanation." Although this might not be what typically comes to mind when we think of abuse, Gallagher goes on to explain: "She left me powerless, impotent, reduced to tears of despair. She herself was renewed in triumph and power . . . By this one act, Miss McGranahan set up problems with sexuality and problems with authority, which I have yet to resolve satisfactorily." Although it is not known exactly how many polio survivors have been abused, certainly many instances have occurred. Statistics on abuse in general are thought to be low because of underreporting by survivors of abuse. This is probably equally true for polio survivors, some of whom are likely to underestimate their life experiences with respect to abuse.

Some individuals may genuinely not have a clear recollection of whether they were abused. More often than not, during the polio epidemics parents and visitors who might potentially protect vulnerable individuals were allowed only very restricted hospital visits. Unlike Gallagher, polio survivors who were children at the time of their hospitalization may not know if or to what extent they were abused. As one female polio survivor told me over lunch, "I'm not sure if I was ever abused, but I remember one vicious nurse who always put the thermometer in the wrong hole." Some readers may find this topic extremely disturbing. I include it here only to point out that issues of former abuse (regardless of whether it was sexual in nature) may contribute to an individual's difficulty in forming loving and physically intimate relationships.

Anyone who has been abused and is still suffering from the effects of that abuse should consider professional help. It could be from a trusted health-care provider, a religious leader, or a psychologist or psychiatrist. Deciding how to go about seeking help will vary for different individuals, and should be done in a way that is most comfortable for the individual.

Post-Polio Syndrome and Sexual Function

Post-Polio Syndrome does not directly cause impotency or sexual dysfunction, although it may indirectly affect sex and intimacy. One of the questions I am asked most often on this topic is whether sex requires too much energy. The answer lies in how important physical intimacy is to a given individual. Certainly having sex requires an expenditure of physical energy. In persons without medical problems, the amount of physical effort required to achieve orgasm (with a familiar partner) is essentially equivalent to walking up a flight of stairs. In polio survivors, walking up a flight of stairs may require much more energy than having sex. If having an intimate relationship is meaningful to you, then the energy expenditure should not preclude your pursuing it.

Remember that *sex does not have to be spontaneous and unplanned.* Adding sex to the list of activities you want to pursue may mean giving up something else in order not to feel overly fatigued. Engaging in sex during the time of day when you have the most energy may help you to enjoy it more and feel less fatigued afterward.

Pain, from PPS or some other cause, may limit sexual desire and pleasure. Treating pain is essential to having a satisfactory quality of life, and any pain that interferes with intimacy should be investigated. Sometimes pain during intercourse can be eliminated simply

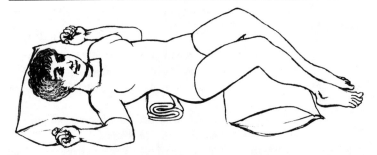

Figure 25.1 For a relatively comfortable position during intercourse, support neck, back, and legs with strategically placed pillows and rolled towels.

by finding a comfortable and supportive position. Figure 25.1 shows how pillows can be used to increase comfort and safety.

How to Handle Problems

If you are having problems with physical intimacy, you should go to your doctor and describe what is happening. A medical doctor is the only individual who has the training necessary to analyze a host of medical illnesses and their possible effects on sexual function combined with the potential side effects of the medications used to treat those conditions. Some problems can be solved in a short office visit, and some may require further evaluation and testing or possibly referral to a specialist. Most doctors are eager to help if people are having problems in these areas, but are reluctant to initiate discussion on such sensitive issues. Therefore, you will probably need to bring up the subject yourself. The majority of physicians understand that intimacy and a satisfying sexual relationship are important parts of most people's lives, regardless of how old they are or whether they have a disability.

The occupational therapist in our clinic initiates discussion with polio survivors by using a modified version of the PLISSIT system, which involves the following steps:[7]

1. *Permission.* The first step is asking the patient for permission to discuss these topics. If the patient is not interested, the subject is dropped. Only at the discretion of the patient do we go any further.
2. *Limited Information.* The next step is to ask for some limited information about the nature of the problems.
3. *Specific Suggestions.* This step involves making suggestions that may involve talking to the doctor about changing medications, trying different positions, and so on.
4. *Intensive Therapy.* For any type of intensive therapy or further diagnostic workup, the patient is referred to a specialist outside the clinic.

Sexual function and intimacy are serious quality-of-life issues for many polio survivors. Health-care providers need to be respectful and pursue these topics only after individuals have indicated their interest in a frank discussion. No one should assume that sex is only for those who are young and able-bodied. Physical intimacy can add a richness to life that nothing else replaces.

CHAPTER 26

Coping with Polio and Post-Polio Syndrome

In his moving book, *When Bad Things Happen to Good People*, Rabbi Harold Kushner writes: "We often find ourselves asking why ordinary people, nice friendly neighbors, neither extraordinarily good nor extraordinarily bad, have to face the agony of pain and tragedy. If the world were fair, they would not seem to deserve it. They are neither very much better nor very much worse than most people we know; why should their lives be so much harder?"[1]

Rabbi Kushner points out what many before him have witnessed: that particularly in the past, people have tried to make sense out of illness and suffering by placing blame on the victims and adopting the attitude that "you get what you deserve." Polio is a perfect example of why this thinking is erroneous and potentially harmful. The most frequent polio victims, incapable of making poor lifestyle choices, were children.

The polio historian and survivor Edmund Sass noted that when the polio epidemics occurred early in the twentieth century, the public's image of persons with disabilities was very negative. In fact, those with physical or mental disabilities were often kept at home with little social interaction—sometimes locked away in a back bedroom. Medical professionals often contributed to this unfortunate perception by labeling people with disabilities "cripples" and treating them dismissively or with disdain. Sass cites one influential orthopedic text published in 1911 that declared, "A failure in the moral training of a cripple means the evolution of an individual detestable in character, a menace and a burden to the community, who is only apt to graduate into the mendicant and criminal classes."[2]

Perhaps one of the most impressive aspects of Franklin Delano Roosevelt's political career was his role in dispelling the long-held myth that persons with disabilities were feeble in mind, body, and character. FDR's famous public-relations campaigns in the face of significant physical adversity provided society with one of the first real glimpses of a disabled man who could succeed with a powerful will and a keen intellect. There is no doubt that FDR did not share the whole of his physical limitations with the public. One particularly memorable episode occurred during the 1936 Democratic national convention when, on his way to the podium, FDR reached out to shake a supporter's hand and suddenly fell, scattering the pages of his speech. Temporarily agitated, he said sharply to his aides, "Clean me up." Roosevelt had established such rapport with the press that no photograph of his fall was ever published and media accounts did not focus on the accident.

Nevertheless, the fact that he was a polio survivor and thus a "cripple" in the eyes of many was enough for history to raise him above his presidential predecessors. FDR, enormously popular and to this day a man whom most historians laud, paved the way for many to live successful lives despite their physical limitations. Indeed, this may have been his most powerful legacy. Yet his image and the way that he handled his life created a double-edged sword for many polio survivors.

Now that the public knew a polio survivor could become one of the most popular presidents of all time, polio survivors felt enormous pressure to become successful too and quite literally to hide any evidence of a physical disability. The focus on being "normal" meant that polio survivors were encouraged to discard as much evidence of their physical limitations as possible. Throwing away crutches, canes, and braces was one of the first steps. Avoidance of clothing that revealed atrophied arms and legs was another unwritten rule. Many polio survivors spent their lifetime trying to perfect a walk without a limp. Others simply avoided situations where their physical limitations might be noticed (such as walking upstairs in front of coworkers).

Frederick Maynard coauthored a commentary on coping styles of polio survivors in which he used the term "passers" to describe polio survivors who went to great lengths to hide their disability from others. Dr. Maynard writes, "By using denial, [polio survivors] have been able to put their disability out of existence mentally and physically and to create an image that completely fools the casual onlooker." He points out, however, that passing requires "constant vigilance to the non-disabled disguise." Polio survivors have lived their lives downplaying and even disguising their disability, often believing that they must continue down this path or they would "blow their cover" and become stigmatized as "handicapped."[3]

To their credit, many polio survivors have done a marvelous job of minimizing their physical disabilities and maximizing their intellectual capabilities. As a group, polio survivors tend to be thought of as successful, hardworking, and intelligent. The point is significant: most polio survivors have not just passed as normal, they have worked extremely hard to let others know that they are capable and competent individuals. It is not surprising, then, that so many polio survivors have attained high levels of achievement both in the workplace and at home.

Jessica Scheer, a respected authority on the attitudes of polio survivors and the social context in which these attitudes are formed, coauthored an article in which she looks at the psychological factors that influence how polio survivors as a group become successful. Scheer writes: "The work ethic had special importance to polio survivors. It was one passage to normalization. The practice of pushing oneself beyond one's limits to achieve goals and 'pass' into the mainstream allowed many persons to not perceive of themselves as handicapped, but simply unable to perform certain functions. The work ethic allowed them to use self-sufficiency, achievement, and productivity as ways to cope with feelings of difference, social rejection, and inequality."[4]

Many polio survivors have consciously or subconsciously repressed feelings of anger, rage, self-pity, and grief in order to move forward and lead successful lives. There are many accounts of polio as a strictly physical ailment with no emotional component. Josephine Walker describes her parents' reaction when she contracted polio as a child: "My parents did everything for me that was needed physically—I was held and carried by my mother for many years. They were in total denial about the fact that there was an emotional component to this. And so they pretended, after a while, like it didn't happen, other than the fact that I needed—you know—a little bit of medical help."[5]

This pattern of ignoring the emotional impact of polio was typical and frequently led to survivors ranking polio as a long-forgotten historical event. The emphasis was on moving forward, not dwelling on how polio affected their lives. However, anyone who survived polio undoubtedly had a significant psychological reaction to this life-altering event, even if those feelings were not expressed. Some polio survivors have used feelings of anger and rage to propel them in their accomplishments. The award-winning author Leonard Kriegel writes on the jacket of his book *Falling into Life*: "It was not the absence of 'normal' legs that fueled my overwhelming sense of anger and loss. My loss was more than physical. And it was certainly not that I had failed to meet the challenge of the polio virus that struck me down when I was eleven. The vanity of a man who has 'overcome a handicap' is formidable. I had earned my survival. And I knew it. But the rage created by loss is more formidable still."[6]

Thus far, I have tried to give the reader a sense of the historical context that impacted the attitudes and coping strategies of many polio survivors. Although not all polio survivors were similarly influenced, it is important to recognize that polio is a chronic illness that will affect individuals in different ways at different times in their lives. Consequently, they will experience a range of emotions as different events occur. Someone experiencing increasing disability will likely feel sad and frustrated, perhaps even angry and depressed. These are normal reactions for people who are dealing with an illness that has the potential to worsen over time.

Over and over I have heard polio survivors describe their grief when they are faced with new problems relating to their old polio. Because they have "conquered" polio once, it seems a cruel trick of nature to be faced with new health problems as a result of having had polio in the past. Nancy Frick has studied the psychological consequences that polio survivors face when they are in this situation. She points out that there are three reasons why polio survivors are particularly vulnerable psychologically when new physical problems arise: (1) they did not know there "was any potential for additional symptoms to occur"; (2) similarly, the medical community was not initially aware that new problems could develop in polio survivors; and (3) polio survivors generally were not in contact with one another, so they had no way of knowing that other polio survivors were experiencing similar difficulties, a fact that often led to social isolation "without medical or emotional support."[7]

We now know polio is not a disease that is "conquered" and never presents another problem; polio survivors may face a host of new issues as they age. However, as Frick points out, the psychological effects of a "second disability" can be "psychologically devastating," particularly in polio survivors who lose the ability to perform certain activities or who experience pain. The grief may be profound and may lead to depression and feelings of worthlessness and despair.

Richard Rossi is an accomplished lawyer in his fifties who contracted polio as a child. He came with his wife to our out-of-town clinic in which polio survivors are evaluated and treated in a concentrated manner over several days. It became apparent to all of us that Richard's wife had urged him to come to the clinic because of her growing concern not only about his physical health, but also about his psychological well-being. At one point she took me aside and confided that she thought Richard was seriously underestimating his grief over his increasing disability. She thought he was depressed and becoming despondent and hopeless. Several months earlier he had made a token suicide attempt, taking a knife and cutting his arms. Unfortunately, Richard had greatly downplayed his sad feelings when he was hospitalized for the suicide attempt, and according to his wife had convinced his doctors to release him with very little follow-up care. He gave the impression of being "a tough old warrior," although he was clearly grieving and depressed when he presented to the polio clinic

Given the magnitude of their afflictions, most polio survivors cope remarkably well. They do experience feelings of frustration and grief, but they find effective ways to deal with them. The explosion of polio support groups around the world is evidence that polio survivors are committed to educating themselves and providing support for others. Still, there are some who become severely depressed. One study found that polio survivors were more likely to become depressed if they were living alone, experiencing new health problems, or had a lot of pain. Depression was also more likely if they were unhappy with their jobs and lacked nurturing relationships with family and friends.[8]

To return to Richard Rossi, he was experiencing new weakness in his legs and arms, and also had a lot of pain. Although he had a loving and supportive wife, he had difficulty communicating his concerns to her and felt that he had to "tough it out." I must emphasize that depression is a treatable illness: both medications and counseling have been shown to be effective. Addressing Richard's depression was a major component of his treatment.

Gerald Sittser is a writer and educator who lost his mother, wife, and young daughter in a tragic car accident. In his memoir, *A Grace Disguised,* Sittser describes his struggle to accept this terrible fate and find value and peace in his life. He writes that although all losses are unique to the individual, there exists a universal experience of loss that we collectively feel as we go through life. "Sooner or later all people suffer loss, in little doses or big ones, suddenly or over time, privately or in public settings. Loss is as much a part of normal life as birth, for as surely as we are born into this world we suffer loss before we leave it."[9]

Sittser points out that loss occurs in two ways, suddenly and unexpectedly or predictably over time. For polio survivors, the loss of their long-standing health status generally occurs fairly predictably over time. Of course, there can be sudden and unexpected losses, as when someone falls and breaks a hip; however, most health issues related to aging with polio do not occur instantaneously.

It is helpful for polio survivors to know this, because it allows them to formulate a plan of action that may include seeking out medical and community support and focusing on lifestyle changes to limit the impact polio will have on them as they age. Polio survivors who are desperate and despondent often feel out of control. They are truly becoming more disabled and have no idea how to slow or stop the process. One of the first things I do in such cases is explain the common ways in which this happens and how to slow or prevent the consequences. In essence, polio is a chronic illness that can take a variety of courses as one ages. Armed with knowledge of how to prevent or minimize future disability, polio survivors become empowered and are able to have some control over their destiny.

Regardless of how vigilant polio survivors are, they will probably still experience some loss of their health status as they age. Sittser points out: "It is not, therefore, the *experience* of loss that becomes the defining moment of our lives, for that is as inevitable as death, which is the last loss awaiting us all. It is how we *respond* to loss that matters. That response will largely determine the quality, the direction, and the impact of our lives."[10]

Cheri Register is a writer and speaker who lives with a rare and incurable liver disease. In her book, *The Chronic Illness Experience*, she writes: "However determined we are to be the arbiters of our own lives, the conviction that we are doing well occasionally falters. Doubts arise especially when our bodies go out of control in spite of our best efforts."[11] Earnest attempts to live a meaningful life filled with patience, optimism, and purpose are impossible to carry out at all times—particularly when health setbacks occur. However, it is a worthwhile goal. Register continues: "How well people manage lives marked by illness depends not on the nature of the illness but on the strength of their conviction that life is worth living no matter what complications are imposed on it . . . Chronic illness, though ever present, is not what matters most in people's lives."[12]

The following coping strategies may be helpful when confronting the spectrum of polio-related issues.

1. *Adapt to having a range of emotions.*

Since polio is a chronic medical condition, polio survivors will go through periods when their health is stable and periods when their health declines. The typical reaction to a decline in physical status is feelings of grief. Thus, a period of mourning is appropriate and expected—regardless of how many times in one's life a decline occurs. Seeking help from professionals (psychiatrists, psychologists, medical social workers) can be beneficial; skilled professionals can help polio survivors cope with the emotional aspects of their chronic illness. Mental health professionals may recommend counseling, medications, or both—not that every polio survivor needs them, but they are available and may be helpful for some people.

2. Accept something less than perfect.

In his book *How Good Do We Have to Be?* Rabbi Harold Kushner addresses the notion that people instinctively strive for perfection. Knowing that perfection is unattainable, he writes, "A lot of misery can be traced to this one mistaken notion: we need to be perfect for people to love us and we forfeit that love if we ever fall short of perfection."[13] Rabbi Kushner goes on to say, "There is a wholeness about the person who has come to terms with his limitations, who knows who he is and what he can and cannot do, the person who has been brave enough to let go of his unrealistic dreams and not feel like a failure for doing so."

3. Take back control.

It is my experience that polio survivors become very anxious when they feel they are losing strength, or they are experiencing pain without the ability to control it. Although it is unrealistic to expect that any of us can completely control what happens to us in the future, polio survivors can take certain measures in order to manage new symptoms and mitigate the severity of future health problems. Polio survivors, more often than not, can positively impact their health and prevent or slow future disability through education, lifestyle changes, and working with experienced health-care providers. Those who are proactive with respect to their physical health will feel more in control and will consequently experience less anxiety and depression.

4. Develop a support network.

In an article on suffering and disability, Barbra Saetersdal notes that "loneliness seems to be the lot of many disabled people."[14] We have seen that people who lack nurturing relationships become more socially isolated and in turn are more susceptible to depression. Friends and family members may not know how to help. They may be worried and confused. Their apparent lack of support may make it seem that they are uncaring or uninterested. Often this is not the case at all. Carol Staudacher suggests adopting the following philosophy: "I will not continue to remain silent. I will give the people who love me a chance to show me their love, to share my pain and for me to share theirs. I will ask for what I need. If I don't get it, I will be no worse off than if I had not asked."[15]

Friends and family are not the only people who can provide support. Clergy are often skilled at counseling. Many polio support groups exist, which are excellent resources for educational materials and support. Going on-line to computer chat rooms may be helpful and allows survivors to express their feelings without necessarily revealing their identity. Regardless of one's approach, a support network can help to avoid the emotional abyss created by social isolation.

Grief, suffering, and loss are present to some degree in everyone's life. There is no need to quantify or compare one person's suffering with another's. We all have our experiences and our reactions to those experiences. Often controlling our destiny really means controlling our reactions. For polio survivors who are faced with new health challenges, addressing the psychological component is just as important as addressing the physical component. As Susan Milstrey Wells writes in *A Delicate Balance*: "Accepting our limitations isn't the same as letting our disease take over our lives . . . Ultimately, acceptance means adapting, more or less gracefully, to the changes that chronic illness brings."[16]

Polio truly is a chronic illness that lasts a lifetime. My hope is that this book will help polio survivors to function at the highest possible levels, both mentally and physically, as they face future health challenges.

Notes

1. Polio—A Look Back

1. J. R. Paul, *History of Poliomyelitis*, New Haven: Yale University Press, 1971.

2. K. Black, *In the Shadow of Polio: A Personal and Social History*, p. 34, New York: Addison Wesley, 1996.

3. N. Rogers, *Dirt and Disease: Polio before FDR*, p. 4, New Brunswick, New Jersey: Rutgers University Press, 1992.

4. E. Tenner, *Why Things Bite Back: Technology and the Revenge of Unintended Consequences*, pp. 56–57, New York: Alfred A. Knopf, 1996.

5. T. Gould, *A Summer Plague: Polio and Its Survivors*, New Haven: Yale University Press, 1995.

6. Ibid., p. 236.

7. E. J. Sass, G. Gottfried, and A. Sorem, eds., *Polio's Legacy: An Oral History*, pp. 33–34, Lanham, Maryland: University Press of America, 1996.

8. L. S. Halstead and G. Grimby, eds., *Post-Polio Syndrome*, pp. 200–1, Philadelphia: Hanley & Belfus, 1995.

9. H. G. Gallagher, *FDR's Splendid Deception: The Moving Story of Roosevelt's Massive Disability and the Intense Efforts to Conceal It from the Public*, 3rd ed., pp. xiii–xiv, Arlington, Virginia: Vandamere Press, 1999.

10. Ibid.

11. Gould, *A Summer Plague*, p. 29.

12. Sass, Gottfried, and Sorem, *Polio's Legacy*.

2. Post-Polio Syndrome

1. L. S. Halstead, ed., *Managing Post-Polio: A Guide to Living Well with Post-Polio Syndrome*, Washington, D.C.: NRH Press, 1998.

2. W. J. W. Sharrard, "The distribution of the permanent paralysis in the lower limb in poliomyelitis," *Journal of Bone and Joint Surgery* 37B (1955): 540–58.

3. L. S. Halstead and J. K. Silver, "Nonparalytic polio and postpolio syndrome," *American Journal of Physical Medicine and Rehabilitation* 79, No. 1 (2000): 13–18.

3. Nonparalytic Polio and Post-Polio Syndrome

1. H. A. Howe and D. Bodian, *Neural Mechanisms of Poliomyelitis,* New York: Commonwealth Fund, 1942; A. B. Sabin and A. J. Steigman, "Poliomyelitis virus of low virulence in patients with epidemic summer grippe or sore throat," *American Journal of Hygiene* 49 (1949): 176–93.

2. L. S. Halstead and J. K. Silver, "Nonparalytic polio and postpolio syndrome," *American Journal of Physical Medicine and Rehabilitation* 79, No. 1 (2000): 13–18.

4. Finding Expert Medical Care

1. G. M. Martin, M. Gordon, and J. J. Opitz, eds., *The First 50 Years,* p. 6, Rochester, Minnesota: American Board of Physical Medicine and Rehabilitation, 1997.

2. Ibid., p. 10.

3. L. A. Leavitt, "Physiatry—both art and science," *Archives of Physical Medicine and Rehabilitation* 48 (1967): 68–70; quotation from p. 68.

4. E. J. Pappert, "Training opportunities for the nineteenth-century American neurologist," *Neurology* 45 (1995): 1771–76; quotations from p. 1772.

5. E. M. Bick, "American orthopedic surgery: I. The first 200 years," *New York State Journal of Medicine* 76 (1976): 1192–97.

6. G. E. Omer, "The development of orthopedic certification in the United States," *Clinical Orthopedics and Related Research* 257 (1990): 11–17.

5. The EMG Controversy

1. A. C. Gawne, B. T. Pham, and L. S. Halstead, "Electrodiagnostic findings in 108 consecutive patients referred to a post-polio clinic: The value of routine electrodiagnostic studies," *Annals of the New York Academy of Sciences* 25 (1995): 383–85.

6. Prevailing over Pain

1. P. Kehret, *Small Steps: The Year I Got Polio,* p. 33, Morton Grove, Illinois: Albert Whitman, 1996.

2. C. Willén and G. Grimby, "Pain, physical activity, and disability in individuals with late effects of polio," *Archives of Physical Medicine and Rehabilitation* 79 (1998): 915–19.

3. L. S. Halstead, ed., *Managing Post-Polio: A Guide to Living Well with Post-Polio Syndrome,* Washington, D.C.: NRH Press, 1998.

8. Sustaining Strength

1. H. Teravainen and D. B. Calne, "Motor system in normal aging and Parkinson's disease," in R. Katzman and R. Terry, eds., *The Neurology of Aging*, pp. 85–109, Philadelphia: F. A. Davis, 1983.

2. A. C. Gawne and L. S. Halstead, "Post-polio syndrome: Pathophysiology and clinical management," *Critical Reviews in Physical and Rehabilitation Medicine* 7 (1995): 147–88.

3. K. Elward and E. B. Larson, "Benefits of exercise for older adults," *Clinics in Geriatric Medicine* 8 (1992): 35–50.

9. Fighting Fatigue

1. P. E. Parsons, *Data on Polio Survivors from the National Health Interview Survey*, Washington, D.C.: National Center for Health Statistics, 1989; R. L. Bruno and N. M. Frick, "Stress and 'type A' behavior as precipitants of post-polio sequelae," in L. S. Halstead and D. O. Wiechers, eds., *Research and Clinical Aspects of the Late Effects of Poliomyelitis*, pp. 145–56, White Plains, New York: March of Dimes, 1987.

2. D. W. Bates, W. Schmitt, D. Buchwald, et al., "Prevalence of fatigue and chronic fatigue syndrome in a primary care practice," *Archives of Internal Medicine* 153 (1993): 2759–65; M. B. Llewelyn, "Assessing the fatigued patient," *British Journal of Hospital Medicine* 55 (1996): 125–29; K. R. Epstein, "The chronically fatigued patient," *Medical Clinics of North America* 79 (1995): 315–27.

3. Parsons, *Data on Polio Survivors*; Bruno and Frick, "Stress and 'type A' behavior."

4. *Taber's Cyclopedic Medical Dictionary*, 15th ed., Philadelphia: F. A. Davis, 1985.

5. R. L. Bruno, R. Sapolsky, J. R. Zimmerman, et al., "Pathophysiology of a central cause of post-polio fatigue," *Annals of the New York Academy of Sciences* 753 (1995): 257–75.

6. R. L. Bruno, N. M. Frick, T. Lewis, et al., "The physiology of post-polio fatigue: A model for post-viral fatigue syndromes and a brain fatigue generator," *CFIDS Chronicle* (1994): 36–42; R. L. Bruno, J. M. Cohen, T. Galski, et al., "The neuroanatomy of post-polio fatigue," *Archives of Physical Medicine and Rehabilitation* 75 (1994): 498–504.

7. J. C. Agre, "Local muscle and total body fatigue," in L. S. Halstead and G. Grimby, eds., *Post-Polio Syndrome*, Philadelphia: Hanley & Belfus, 1995.

8. J. R. Bach and A. S. Alba, "Pulmonary dysfunction and sleep disordered breathing as post-polio sequelae: Evaluation and management," *Orthopedics* 14 (1991): 1329–37.

9. R. L. Bruno, J. R. Zimmerman, S. J. Creange, et al., "Bromocriptine in the treatment of post-polio fatigue," *American Journal of Physical Medicine and Rehabilitation* 75 (1996): 340–47.

10. Controlling Cold Intolerance

1. D. A. Campbell and S. P. Kay, "What is cold intolerance?" *Journal of Hand Surgery (British and European)* 23B (1998): 3−5.

2. L. S. Halstead, ed., *Managing Post-Polio: A Guide to Living Well with Post-Polio Syndrome*, Washington, D.C.: NRH Press, 1998.

3. S. M. Macey and D. F. Schneider, "Deaths from excessive heat and excessive cold among the elderly," *Gerontologist* 33 (1993): 497−500.

11. Respiratory Problems

1. J. R. Bach and A. S. Alba, "Pulmonary dysfunction and sleep disordered breathing as post-polio sequelae: Evaluation and management," *Orthopedics* 14 (1991): 1329−37; "Pathophysiology of paralytic-restrictive pulmonary syndromes," in J. R. Bach, ed., *Pulmonary Rehabilitation: The Obstruction and Paralytic Conditions*, pp. 275−83, Philadelphia: Hanley & Belfus, 1996.

2. K. Borg and L. Kaijser, "Lung function in patients with prior poliomyelitis," *Clinical Physiology* 10 (1990): 201−12; D. Kidd, R. S. Howard, A. J. Williams, et al., "Late functional deterioration following paralytic poliomyelitis," *Quarterly Journal of Medicine* 90 (1997): 189−96.

3. A. C. Dean, B. A. Graham, M. Dalakas, et al., "Sleep apnea in patients with postpolio syndrome," *Annals of Neurology* 43 (1998): 661−64; A. A. Hsu and B. A. Staats, " 'Postpolio' sequelae and sleep-related disordered breathing," *Mayo Clinic Proceedings* 73 (1998): 216−24.

4. Bach, "Pathophysiology of paralytic-restrictive pulmonary syndromes."

5. J. W. Choi, T. R. Saunders, O. Tebrock, et al., "Comparison of different mechanical ventilators for patients with poliomyelitis," *Military Medicine* 160 (1995): 293−96; J. R. Bach and A. S. Alba, "Management alternatives for postpolio respiratory insufficiency: Assisted ventilation by nasal or oral-nasal interface," *American Journal of Physical Medicine and Rehabilitation* 68 (1989): 264−71.

6. G-F. W. Yang, A. Alba, M. Lee, et al., "Pneumobelt for sleep in the ventilator user: Clinical experience," *Archives of Physical Medicine and Rehabilitation* 70 (1989): 707−11; C. Iber, S. F. Davies, and M. W. Mahowald, "Nocturnal rocking bed therapy: Improvement in sleep fragmentation in patients with respiratory muscle weakness," *Sleep* 12 (1989): 405−12; "Conventional approaches to managing neuromuscular ventilatory failure," in J. R. Bach, ed., *Pulmonary Rehabilitation: The Obstruction and Paralytic Conditions*, pp. 285−301, Philadelphia: Hanley & Belfus, 1996.

7. T. R. Harrison and A. S. Fauci, in A. S. Fauci, E. Braunwald, K. J. Isselbacher, et al., eds., *Harrison's Principles of Internal Medicine*, 14th ed., New York: McGraw-Hill, 1998.

8. Dean, Graham, Dalakas, et al., "Sleep apnea in patients with postpolio syndrome."

9. Harrison and Fauci, *Harrison's Principles of Internal Medicine.*

12. Swallowing Issues

1. L. R. Robinson, A. D. Hillel, and P. F. Waugh, "New laryngeal muscle weakness in post-polio syndrome," *Laryngoscope* 108 (1998): 732–34; B. P. Driscoll, C. Gracco, C. Coelho, et al., "Laryngeal function in postpolio patients," *Laryngoscope* 105 (1995): 35–41; K. M. Nugent, "Vocal cord paresis and glottic stenosis: A late complication of poliomyelitis," *South Medical Journal* 80 (1987): 1594–95.

2. C. A. Coelho and R. Ferranti, "Incidence and nature of dysphagia in polio survivors," *Archives of Physical Medicine and Rehabilitation* 72 (1991): 1071–75.

3. M. Dowhaniuk and C. T. Schentag, "Dysphagia in individuals with no history of bulbar polio," *Annals of the New York Academy of Sciences* 753 (1995): 405–7.

4. B. Ivanyi, S. K. Saffire, S. Phoa, and M. de Visser, "Dysphagia in postpolio patients: A videofluorographic follow-up study," *Dysphagia* 9 (1994): 96–98; B. C. Sonies, "Dysphagia and post-polio syndrome: Past, present, and future," *Seminars in Neurology* 6 (1996): 365–70.

5. B. Gustafsson and L. Tibbling, "Dysphagia, an unrecognized handicap," *Dysphagia* 6 (1991): 193–99.

6. W. G. Paterson, "Dysphagia in the elderly," *Canadian Family Physician* 42 (1996): 925–32.

7. S. Lindgren and L. Janzon, "Prevalence of swallowing complaints and clinical findings among 50–79 year-old men and women in an urban population," *Dysphagia* 6 (1991): 187–92.

8. M. Broniatowski, B. C. Sonies, J. S. Rubin, et al., "Current evaluation and treatment of patients with swallowing disorders," *Otolaryngological Head and Neck Surgery* 120 (1999): 464–73.

13. Exercise Essentials

1. J. C. Agre, "The role of exercise in the patient with post-polio syndrome," *Annals of the New York Academy of Sciences* 753 (1995): 321–34.

2. H. Gallagher, "The loneliness of the long-distance runner," *Greater Boston Post-Polio Association (Triumph)* (Fall 1996): 1. Reprinted from *New Mobility*.

3. H. S. Milner-Brown, "Muscle strengthening in a post-polio subject through a high-resistance weight-training program," *Archives of Physical Medicine and Rehabilitation* 74 (1993): 1165–67; S. A. Spector, P. L. Gordon, I. M. Feuerstein, et al., "Strength gains without muscle injury after strength training in patients with postpolio muscular atrophy," *Muscle and Nerve* 19 (1996): 1282–90; J. C. Agre, A. A. Rodriguez, and T. M. Franke, "Strength, endurance, and work capacity after muscle strengthening exercise in postpolio subjects," *Archives of Physical Medicine and Rehabilitation* 78 (1997): 681–86; J. C. Agre, A. A. Rodriguez, T. M. Franke, et al., "Low-intensity, alternate-day exercise improves

muscle performance without apparent adverse effect in postpolio patients," *American Journal of Physical Medicine and Rehabilitation* 75 (1996): 50–58; M. J. Fillyaw, G. J. Badger, G. D. Goodwin, et al., "Post-polio sequelae: The effects of long-term non-fatiguing resistance exercise in subjects with post-polio syndrome," *Orthopedics* 14 (1991): 1253–56.

4. L. S. Halstead, A. C. Gawne, and B. T. Pham, "National Rehabilitation Hospital limb classification for exercise, research, and clinical trials in postpolio patients," *Annals of the New York Academy of Sciences* 753 (1995): 343–53.

5. U.S. Department of Health and Human Services, *Physical Activity and Health: A Report of the Surgeon General,* p. 6, Pittsburgh: U.S. Department of Health and Human Services, 1996.

6. K. Elward and E. B. Larson, "Benefits of exercise for older adults," *Health Promotion and Disease Prevention* 8 (1992): 35–50.

7. R. R. Owen and D. Jones, "Polio residuals clinic: Conditioning exercise program," *Orthopedics* 8 (1985): 882–83.

8. American Heart Association, *Heart and Stroke Statistical Update,* Dallas: American Heart Association, 1997.

9. National Institute of Diabetes and Digestive and Kidney Diseases (NIH), *Diabetes Statistics,* U.S. Department of Health and Human Services, 1995.

10. Edward and Larson, "Benefits of exercise for older adults."

11. R. R. Yeung, "The acute effects of exercise on mood state," *Journal of Psychosomatic Research* 40 (1996): 123–41.

14. Energy Conservation and Pacing

1. H. G. Gallagher, "Growing old with polio: A personal perspective," in L. S. Halstead and G. Grimby, eds., *Post-Polio Syndrome,* p. 218, Philadelphia: Hanley & Belfus, 1995.

2. D. Christy and C. A. Sarafconn, *Pacing Yourself: Steps to Help Save Your Energy,* p. viii, Bloomington, Illinois: Cheever Publishing, 1990.

3. D. L. Goldenberg, *Chronic Illness and Uncertainty: A Personal and Professional Guide to Poorly Understood Syndromes,* p. 76, Newton Lower Falls, Massachusetts: Dorset Press, 1996.

16. Preventing Falls and Further Disability

1. K. K. Steinweg, "The changing approach to falls in the elderly," *American Family Physician* 56 (1997): 1815–22.

2. G. M. Tibbitts, "Patients who fall: How to predict and prevent injuries," *Geriatrics* 51 (1996): 24–31.

3. T. M. Cutson, "Falls in the elderly," *American Family Physician* 49 (1994): 149–56.

4. R. Tideiksaar, "Preventing falls: How to identify risk factors, reduce complications," *Geriatrics* 51 (1996): 43–53.

5. E. B. Wilson, "Preventing patient falls," *AACN Clinical Issues* 9 (1998):

100–8; A. J. Campbell, M. C. Robertson, and M. M. Gardner, "Elderly people who fall: Identifying and managing the causes," *British Journal of Hospital Medicine* 54 (1995): 520–23.

6. R. W. Sattin, J. G. Rodriguez, C. A. DeVito, et al., "Home environmental hazards and the risk of fall injury events among community-dwelling older persons," *Journal of the American Geriatrics Society* 46 (1998): 669–76; J. G. Rodriguez, A. L. Baughman, R. W. Sattin, et al., "A standardized instrument to assess hazards for falls in the home of older persons," *Accident, Analysis and Prevention* 27 (1995): 625–31.

7. W. P. Berg, H. M. Alessio, E. M. Mills, et al., "Circumstances and consequences of falls in independent community-dwelling older adults," *Age and Ageing* 26 (1997): 261–68; quotation from p. 261.

8. D. Hemenway, S. J. Solnick, C. Koeck, et al., "The incidence of stairway injuries in Austria," *Accident, Analysis and Prevention* 26 (1994): 674–79.

9. Steinweg, "The changing approach to falls in the elderly."

10. R. G. Cumming, "Epidemiology of medication-related falls and fractures in the elderly," *Drugs and Aging* 12 (1998): 43–53; M. Monane and J. Avorn, "Medications and falls: Causation, correlation, and prevention," *Clinics in Geriatric Medicine* 12 (1996): 847–58.

11. E. Dean and J. Ross, "Relationships among cane fitting, function, and falls," *Physical Therapy* 73 (1993): 494–504.

17. Keeping Bones Healthy and Strong

1. National Osteoporosis Foundation, *Osteoporosis: Physician's Guide to Prevention and Treatment of Osteoporosis*, Belle Mead, New Jersey: Excerpta Medica, 1998.

2. J. G. Haddad, "Osteoporosis in men," *Revue du Rheumatisme* [English ed.] 64 (1997): 81S–83S.

3. J. D. Ringe, "Hip fractures in men," *Osteoporosis International* 3 Supplement (1996): S48–S51; E. Seeman, "Osteoporosis in men," *Baillière's Clinical Rheumatology* 11 (1997): 613–29.

4. National Osteoporosis Foundation, *Osteoporosis*, jacket.

5. T. M. Cutson, "Falls in the elderly," *American Family Physician* 49 (1994): 149–56.

6. R. Tideiksaar, "Preventing falls: How to identify risk factors, reduce complications," *Geriatrics* 51 (1996): 43–53; M. E. Tinetti and M. Speechley, "Prevention of falls among the elderly," *New England Journal of Medicine* 320 (1989): 1055–59; K. K. Steinweg, "The changing approach to falls in the elderly," *American Family Physician* 56 (1997): 1815–22.

7. C. L. Deal, "Osteoporosis: Prevention, diagnosis, and management," *American Journal of Medicine* 102 Supplement (1997): 35S–39S; P. T. Packard and R. P. Heaney, "Medical nutrition therapy for patients with osteoporosis," *Journal of the American Diet Association* 97 (1997): 414–17; K. O. O'Brien, "Com-

bined calcium and vitamin D supplementation reduces bone loss and fracture incidence in older men and women," *Nutrition Reviews* 56 (1998): 148–58.

8. E. Seeman, "Osteoporosis: Trials and tribulations," *American Journal of Medicine* 103 (1997): 74S–89S.

18. Mobility

1. A. E. Minetti, C. Capelli, P. Zamparo, et al., "Effects of stride frequency on mechanical power and energy expenditure of walking," *Medicine and Science in Sports and Exercise* 27 (1995): 1194–1202; K. G. Holt, J. Hamill, and R. O. Andres, "Predicting the minimal energy costs of human walking," *Medicine and Science in Sports and Exercise* 23 (1991): 491–98; P. J. Corcoran, R. H. Jebsen, G. L. Brengelmann, et al., "Effects of plastic and metal leg braces on speed and energy cost of hemiparetic ambulation," *Archives of Physical Medicine and Rehabilitation* 51 (1970): 69–77; H. B. Skinner and R. L. Barrack, "Ankle weighting effect on gait in able-bodied adults," *Archives of Physical Medicine and Rehabilitation* 71 (1990): 112–15.

2. S. L. Barnett, A. M. Bagley, and H. B. Skinner, "Ankle weight effect on gait: Orthotic implications," *Orthopedics* 16 (1993): 1127–31; W. P. Waring, F. Maynard, W. Grady, et al., "Influence of appropriate lower extremity orthotic management on ambulation, pain, and fatigue in a postpolio population," *Archives of Physical Medicine and Rehabilitation* 70 (1989): 371–75.

3. M. P. Foley, B. Prax, R. Crowell, et al., "Effects of assistive devices on cardiorespiratory demands in older adults," *Physical Therapy* 76 (1996): 1313–19.

4. G. D. Foster, T. A. Wadden, Z. V. Kendrick, et al., "The energy cost of walking before and after significant weight loss," *Medicine and Science in Sports and Exercise* 27 (1995): 888–94.

5. J. Perry, S. J. Mulroy, and S. E. Renwick, "The relationship of lower extremity strength and gait parameters in patients with post-polio syndrome," *Archives of Physical Medicine and Rehabilitation* 74 (1993): 165–69; J. Perry, J. D. Fontaine, and S. Mulroy, "Findings in post-poliomyelitis syndrome," *Journal of Bone and Joint Surgery* 77-A (1995): 1148–53.

19. Bracing, Shoes and Assistive Devices

1. J. K. Silver, D. D. Aiello, and R. Drillio, "Lightweight carbon fiber and kevlar floor reaction AFO in two polio survivors with new weakness," *Archives of Physical Medicine and Rehabilitation* 80 (1999): 1180; M. Heim, E. Yaacobi, and M. Azaria, "A pilot study to determine the efficiency of lightweight carbon fibre orthoses in the management of patients suffering from post-poliomyelitis syndrome, *Clinical Rehabilitation* 11 (1997): 302–5.

20. Wheelchairs and Scooters

1. R. Woods, *Tales from inside the Iron Lung and How I Got out of It*, p. 24, Philadelphia: University of Pennsylvania Press, 1994.

22. Complementary and Alternative Medicine

1. Risk Management Foundation, "Complementary and alternative medicine (CAM)," in P. B. Martin and H. Groff, eds., *Forum* 19, No. 6 (1999): 1–13. Reprinted from National Institutes of Health; quotation from p. 1.

2. "Acupuncture," *NIH Consensus Statement* 15, No. 5 (1997): 1–34.

3. C. Vallbona, C. F. Hazlewood, and G. Jurida, "Response of pain to static magnetic fields in postpolio patients: A double-blind pilot study," *Archives of Physical Medicine and Rehabilitation* 78 (1997): 1200–3.

23. Designing a Safe and Comfortable Living Environment

1. J. Aird, "Remodeling: Where to get financial help when modifying your home," *Accent on Living* (1998): 58–65.

2. B. Garee, ed., *Ideas for Making Your Home Accessible,* Bloomington, Illinois: Cheever Publishing, 1994; R. Cheever and B. Garee, eds., *An Accent Guide: An Accessible Home of Your Own,* Bloomington, Illinois: Cheever Publishing, 1990.

3. See L. H. Trachtman, ed., *Assistive Technology,* Arlington, Virginia: RESNA Press, 1998.

24. Insurance and Disability Benefits

1. In L. S. Halstead, ed., *Managing Post-Polio: A Guide to Living Well with Post-Polio Syndrome,* p. 216, Washington, D.C.: NRH Press, 1998.

2. E. J. Sass, G. Gottfried, and A. Sorem, eds., *Polio's Legacy: An Oral History,* p. 239, Lanham, Maryland: University Press of America, 1996.

25. Sex and Intimacy

1. W. S. Woodard and S. A. Rollin, "Sexuality and the elderly: Obstacles and options," *Journal of Rehabilitation* 47 (1981): 64–68; F. E. Kaiser, "Sexuality in the elderly," *Urologic Clinics of North America* 23 (1996): 99–109.

2. C. Eliopoulos, *Gerontological Nursing,* 4th ed., p. 207, Philadelphia: Lippincott, 1997.

3. D. C. Renshaw, "Sexual problems in old age, illness, and disability," *Psychosomatics* 22 (1981): 975–85.

4. E. M. Dagon, "Problems and prospects with sexuality and aging," *Wisconsin Medical Journal* 80 (1981): 37–39; Geriatrics panel discussion, "Sexual problems in the elderly, I: The use and abuse of medications," *Geriatrics* 44 (1989): 61–71.

5. K. Hwang, "Living with a disability: A woman's perspective," in M. L. Sipski and C. J. Alexander, eds., *Sexual Function in People with Disability and Chronic Illness,* p. 119, Gaithersburg, Maryland: Aspen Publishers, 1997.

6. H. G. Gallagher, *Black Bird Fly Away: Disabled in an Able-Bodied World,* p. 46, Arlington, Virginia: Vandamere Press, 1998.

7. J. S. Annon, *The Behavioral Treatment of Sexual Problems: Brief Therapy*, New York: Harper and Row, 1976.

26. Coping with Polio and Post-Polio Syndrome

1. H. S. Kushner, *When Bad Things Happen to Good People*, p. 8, New York: Avon Books, 1981.

2. E. J. Sass, G. Gottfried, and A. Sorem, eds., *Polio's Legacy: An Oral History*, p. 7, Lanham, Maryland: University Press of America, 1996.

3. F. M. Maynard and S. Roller, "Recognizing typical coping styles of polio survivors can improve rehabilitation," *American Journal of Physical Medicine and Rehabilitation*, 70 (1991): 70–72; quotation from p. 70.

4. J. Scheer and M. L. Luborsky, "Post-polio sequelae: The cultural context of polio biographies," *Orthopedics* 14 (1991): 1173–81; quotation from p. 1178.

5. T. Gould, *A Summer Plague: Polio and Its Survivors*, p. 102, New Haven: Yale University Press, 1995.

6. L. Kriegel, *Falling into Life: Essays*, San Francisco: North Point Press, 1991.

7. N. M. Frick, "Post-polio sequelae and the psychology of second disability," *Orthopedics* 8 (1985): 851–53; quotation from pp. 851–52.

8. D. Tate, N. Kirsch, F. Maynard, et al., "Coping with the late effects: Differences between depressed and nondepressed polio survivors," *American Journal of Physical Medicine and Rehabilitation* 73 (1994): 27–35.

9. G. L. Sittser, *A Grace Disguised: How the Soul Grows through Loss*, p. 9, Grand Rapids, Michigan: Zondervan Publishing House, 1995.

10. Ibid.

11. C. Register, *The Chronic Illness Experience: Embracing the Imperfect Life*, p. xix, Center City, Minnesota: Hazelden, 1987.

12. Ibid., p. xxii.

13. H. S. Kushner, *How Good Do We Have to Be?*, pp. 9, 179, Boston: Little, Brown, 1996.

14. B. Saetersdal, "Forbidden suffering: The Pollyanna syndrome of the disabled and their families," *Family Process, Inc.* 36 (1997): 431–35; quotation from p. 434.

15. C. Staudacher, *A Time to Grieve: Meditations for Healing after the Death of a Loved One*, p. 164, San Francisco: Harper, 1994.

16. S. M. Wells, *A Delicate Balance: Living Successfully with Chronic Illness*, pp. 158, 160, Reading, Massachusetts: Perseus Books, 1998.

Index